Natural Curly Hair

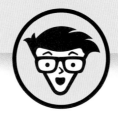

Natural & Curly Hair

by Johnny Wright
Celebrity Hair Stylist
FOREWORD BY Tamron Hall, Host and
Executive Producer and Host, *Tamron Hall Show*

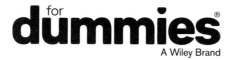

for
dummies®
A Wiley Brand

Natural & Curly Hair For Dummies®

Published by: **John Wiley & Sons, Inc.,** 111 River Street, Hoboken, NJ 07030-5774, www.wiley.com

For general information on our other products and services, please contact our Customer Care Department within the U.S. at 877-762-2974, outside the U.S. at 317-572-3993, or fax 317-572-4002. For technical support, please visit www.wiley.com/techsupport.

Wiley publishes in a variety of print and electronic formats and by print-on-demand. Some material included with standard print versions of this book may not be included in e-books or in print-on-demand. If this book refers to media such as a CD or DVD that is not included in the version you purchased, you may download this material at http://booksupport.wiley.com. For more information about Wiley products, visit www.wiley.com.

Library of Congress Control Number: 2022945759

ISBN: 978-1-119-84338-2 (pbk); ISBN: 978-1-119-84339-9 (ebk); ISBN: 978-1-119-84340-5 (ebk)

Contents at a Glance

Table of Contents

Foreword

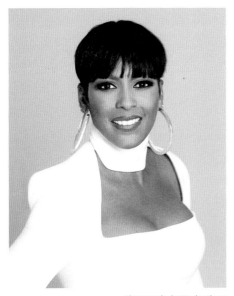

Photography by Kwaku Alston

t's fair to say Johnny Wright never gets it wrong. I say that with great confidence because I know, firsthand, that when it comes to hair, Johnny puts his heart into every strand. That's because hair is truly in his blood.

The grandson of a hairstylist, Johnny's relationship with hair started at birth. He embraces how important our hair is to our identities and how we express ourselves. And when it comes to natural hair, Johnny knows that the topic is fraught and hits so many nerves. It can also be a source of insecurity. But when you embrace your natural look, you can inspire and you can feel confident. Your hair — and especially your natural hair — can even be a statement, perhaps a political statement.

Regardless of how you choose to wear it, this book will teach you how to care for your hair and your heart at the same time. Johnny has taught me — and a long list of clients, celebrity and layperson alike — that these two things are connected.

After many years in the business, after so much research and so many conversations, Johnny understands the wants and needs of people looking for answers on how to properly care for their natural hair. His advice is approachable and accessible because that's how he was raised. The roots!

This book is about making sure that your crown is on straight and everyone can see the glory that comes when you feel good about your hair.

Few others could offer such a textured journey with tips on each page to make your life a little easier. Read on to ensure every curl, coil, wave, and spiral is healthy and beautiful and unapologetically natural — like Johnny Wright.

—Tamron Hall

Introduction

Whether you're here for yourself or someone you love, welcome! At first glance, this might look like a book. But to me, it's so much more than that. What you hold in your hands is your space. It's your place. It's a living, breathing community of people coming together to understand, to heal, and to live life to the fullest.

Within these pages, you can find creation, inspiration, and celebration of our natural and curly hair community. This book lays out everything you need to know to care for healthy textured hair and figure out how to style it like the star it is. You don't have to do hours of web searches to find styling tutorials or get stacks of books that each have one little chapter on natural hair maintenance. On the contrary, this book has everything you need to get started on the right path. It's all about your hair care needs.

From cover to cover, this book is filled with how-to's, professional hairstylist tips, product recommendations, and so much more — and it's all (and only) for natural and curly hair. Forget about having only one small paragraph dedicated to natural and curly hair, like an afterthought, in a hair care book.

In this book, we explore the complex beauty of what natural and curly hair really means. I go beyond what you see on your head, and I talk about all the ways your hair connects to your heart and soul. They say that beauty is only skin deep, but to me, beauty is really about how you can reflect your power in all aspects of yourself, including your hair. Be who you truly are without hiding or feeling shame. And the natural and curly hair community has had a tough fight.

With this book, I'm here to help build you up, nurture you, and help you embrace your God-given beauty in all its glory. If you've spent one second not feeling like the radiant being you are because of your hair, that's one second too many.

This is a new beginning for you and for me — for us. We're sharing a very important journey, and I couldn't be happier and prouder to be here with you.

And one final note before we really dive in: I've done my very best to pack this book full of something for everyone, but there's so much to say, I could write a whole library on this subject! So, in some places, I give you my recommendations for additional resources and places to go for more support and help.

I hope you're as excited about reading this book as I am writing it. It's long overdue, and I'm so happy to bring this to you. It's all about curl power!

If you or someone you love has natural and curly hair, you've come to the right place. You hold in your hands a book that's chock-full of everything you need to know about keeping curly and natural hair healthy, styling it the way you want, and most of all, celebrating it every day in every way!

This book centers the spotlight on natural and curly hair within the African Diaspora (Black, Afro-Latinidad, and biracial) to address specific topics about hair care and styling within those communities. In this book, I not only give you the nuts and bolts of tools, products, and step-by-step instructions, but also provide some inspiration, motivation, and full support so that you can unlock the magic and beauty of your natural and curly hair.

Whether you've flaunted your curls your whole life and are looking for some new ideas to freshen up your look; you're transitioning away from relaxed hair to fully natural; or you have a child or other loved one who's blessed with beautifully textured hair that you want to figure out how to care for — this book is here to support your amazing hair journey, from root to tip.

About This Book

Although you can find a few hair care books and plenty online tutorials out there, this book is different. It brings together everything you need to know to live your best curly and natural hair life. This book gives you a little history on the power and journey of natural hair, little bits of basic hair biology info, insider pro tips for the best products and tools, and step-by-step processes for all the essential styles — from braids, to twists, to afros, and for those who love to heat style their hair. This book isn't just one thing for one person; it's textured and layered, just like the hair it celebrates. It's part instruction manual, part personal shopper, part style maven, and *allllll* about you.

Like all *For Dummies* books, the formatting of this book makes it super easy for you to find the information you want quickly and at a glance. To make the content more accessible, I divided it into six parts.

In Part 1, I set the stage for you so you can fully understand your unique head of hair. Go here if you want to explore anatomy and the science of your locs. In Part 2, I go over all the routines and regular maintenance you need to do to keep your hair healthy. If you want help with your daily routines or weekly wash days, this is the part for you. In Part 3, I take you through the land of products and tools so you can select the supplies that are best for you. If you need help making sense of your shopping options, this is where to go. In Part 4, I guide you as you discover how to do different styles. This is the part you need if you want to rock a certain look. In Part 5, I give you the lowdown on how to care for kids' hair. This part is made just for parents, guardians, and all adults who care for kids with natural and curly hair. Finally, in Part 6, I give you some extra bonus content and also boil down the book into very small chunks of information. Go here if you need quick info right away.

Disclaimer: The reader should note that the author of this publication has a paid partnership with RevAir LLC (RevAir) and PDC Brands (Cantu) and a partnership with Techturized, Inc. (Myavana) to promote their respective brands and products on social media, television, and other media sources. The author lists some brands and products from those companies in this book as some of his favorite products.

Icons Used in This Book

Throughout this book, icons in the margins highlight certain types of valuable information that call out for your attention. Here are the icons you encounter and a brief description of each:

The Tip icon calls out bits of insider info you can use to make your hair care easy and extra amazing. It's like having your own personal hairstylist whispering their best pro tips in your ear.

Remember icons mark the information that's especially important to know. If you don't have time to read anything else, look for these icons. They contain all of the must-know stuff.

If I mark something with this icon, the information I give may help you go to the next level in your quest for hair knowledge. But you don't have to read paragraphs marked with this icon unless you really want to get into the nitty gritty of hair care.

The Warning icon tells you to watch out! Always read whatever information features this icon because it keeps you and your hair safe. This icon calls out things that you should do or shouldn't do to make sure you don't damage your (or someone else's) hair.

Beyond the Book

In addition to the abundance of natural and curly hair information and guidance that I provide in this book, you get access to even more help and information online at Dummies.com. Check out this book's online Cheat Sheet for quick info on how to grow out your natural hair, to see a list of the most essential styling tools and products, DIY hair care recipes, and more. Just go to www.dummies.com and search for "Natural and Curly Hair For Dummies Cheat Sheet."

Where to Go from Here

Like I said, this book has something for everyone — which means it probably has something that you don't need. But the great news is that you don't have to read everything. *For Dummies* books are modular, which means each part and the different chapters can stand alone. You don't have to read the early chapters to understand the later ones. Skip around and go directly to the information you need without wasting time reading stuff you don't.

If, for example, you're caring for a child who's having a hair emergency right now and you need to know how to do a simple ponytail or braids, flip to Chapter 12. If you just need some help picking new products and tools that work for you and your hair, head over to Chapters 7 and 8. If you're wondering what changes to make to your daily routine to keep your natural and curly hair its happiest, turn to Chapter 5. And if you're curious about the history, biology, and other basics of natural and curly hair, start with Chapters 1 and 2. So let's get your natural hair journey started!

1

Embracing Your Natural and Curly Hair

IN THIS PART . . .

Appreciate the history, beauty, and power of natural and curly hair.

Grasp the basics of hair biology.

Uncover your hair type profile and its characteristics.

Chapter **1**

Natural Is Beautiful

This chapter is about helping you feel your absolute best. That's all that matters, as far as I'm concerned. Your hair is an extension of your personality, your energy, your heart. I want you to be able to take care of your hair and style it in all the ways that make you feel like your best self — or help you do that for someone else. This chapter can help you have the healthiest hair possible, as well as the best relationship with your hair.

There are so many reasons we can feel negatively about our hair. People with curly, natural hair have not been seen as a thing of beauty for so long. Black women especially have been conditioned and treated like they are unattractive for having natural hair, and some women have internalized this hatred and adjusted their hair accordingly. A client of mine recently pointed out how she and her close friends often feel great pressure to process and straighten their hair due to their experience with men and dating and other negative influences within the community. So many men have been conditioned to want and be attracted to a particular representation of beauty because of the relentless standards set by the media. We have seen straight hair put out as the normal, acceptable standard for so long that it's shaped entire generations. This, too, is trauma.

Unhealthy beauty standards have been ingrained in Western culture by systems underpinned by totally toxic ideas. But the time has come to heal. You need to reclaim your power and your beauty, and move beyond self-hatred. Refuse to buy into the toxicity. Refuse the negativity and trauma.

This chapter promotes being really honest about who you are and only surrounding yourself with people who see you, support you, and celebrate you. This is your moment. This is the natural and curly haired community's moment to step into the spotlight.

Smashing the Stigma Surrounding Natural Hair

Okay, look. I don't want to spend time and energy on what the natural and curly hair community has or doesn't have. I'm here to focus on building our community up, to help lift us up. That's how we celebrate ourselves.

But the truth is the truth. Those of us who have natural hair already know it. But maybe you're someone who doesn't have textured hair and you're reading this book to understand a loved one. If you don't already know, people who have natural and curly hair regularly face discrimination, misunderstandings, and misconceptions about their hair, all based in centuries-old racism that plays out in media, workplaces, and schools, among other institutions.

Unfortunately, you can find so many examples of the systemic discrimination that Black and Afro-Latinidad people who have natural hair face. One national news story that absolutely enraged me when I saw it back in 2019 still stays with me today. Before his wrestling match, a 16-year-old high school student in New Jersey was told by officials that his hair covering didn't meet "regulation standards." They presented him with an ultimatum: Cut his dreads or forfeit the match. Without so much as a word from his coach, the athletic director, or any other staff member from his school, he faced the decision alone.

And there, in front of a whole gymnasium of his peers and members of the community, an official cut off his dreadlocks. He went on to win the wrestling match that day, but the humiliation of having his hair carelessly cut off due to policies that do not represent everyone equally may never fade.

This student's natural state of being was deemed unacceptable and deserving of immediate destruction. And this scenario, in some form or another, plays out in schools and workplaces across the country, literally every day.

How dare they perpetuate this level of hatred and trauma on children — and adults!

The natural and curly hair community faces unfair treatment and downright stupidity from some people and systems. Because these prejudices are so deeply ingrained, society as a whole can find even recognizing them difficult, let alone combating them.

But I'm not going to stop trying. I'm here with this book to do my part in stopping the stigma; in building the natural and curly hair community up; in saying enough to the discrimination from others and the way we internalize it ourselves.

It's time to stop. And it's time to heal. And that means everyone.

So, if you need support in your own healing journey, you have it here. And if you're a parent of a textured-haired child, you need to know the reality of prejudices and racism, and then smash this stigma for your child (or other loved one). Natural and curly hair is beautiful and glorious (see Figure 1-1).

From the moment your child who has textured hair is born (or the moment you become their guardian), celebrate their beautiful hair at every turn. I talk more about how to be your child's hair advocate in Chapter 11, but that advice is good for all ages.

And if you have natural hair — or you want to wear your hair in its natural state but are fighting against these negative forces — then I'm here to tell you something:

They might be powerful, but you are more powerful!

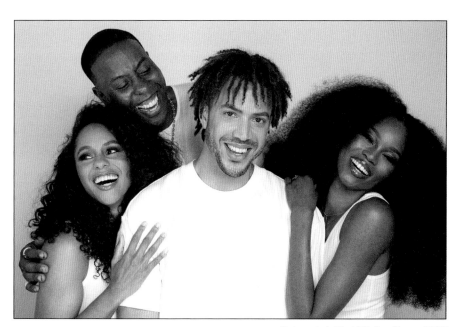

FIGURE 1-1:
Natural
and curly hair
is versatile
and beautiful.

Photography by Wardell Malloy with crowdMGMT

Laying the naysayers to rest

I don't want to give any attention to the myths that people hold onto, especially because we've all dealt with combating them. And frankly, if someone continues to hold onto anything negative, that's on them.

My best advice is to not pay any attention to people who have anything negative or misinformed to say about natural and curly hair. Of course, if you want to engage and educate others — particularly if they're coming from a place of honest ignorance — that's up to you. But my personal advice is to not even waste your time or energy with anyone who's willfully ignorant or just plain rude.

The best way to lay any myths to rest is to go out and live your best, happiest hair life. Don't listen to anyone who says you or your child can't do something with your or their hair. Don't listen to anyone who tries to make you or your child feel inferior. Never forget that textured hair grows beautifully out of the scalp the way it's meant to.

Embracing today's changing attitudes

Attitudes toward hair texture are gradually changing for the better. Natural hair is seeing a golden age right now, where it's represented and presented in the proper light. More products and tools specifically for natural and curly hair are available in retail stores nationwide.

Even while the media celebrates and spotlights others copying natural hairstyles, the bias still persists. I mean, we still see stories in the news on the regular that report about school officials not allowing students to wear natural or protective styles, like the one I share in the section "Smashing the Stigma Surrounding Natural Hair," earlier in this chapter.

But you can also see individual and mass efforts — amplified by social and other broadcast media — to dismantle these discriminatory policies.

At the forefront of a legislative effort is the CROWN Act, created by the CROWN Coalition and passed into law first in the state of California in 2019. CROWN stands for *Creating a Respectful and Open World for Natural Hair.* The CROWN Act works to "ensure protection against discrimination towards race-based hairstyles by extending statutory protection to hair texture and protective styles, such as braids, locs, twists, and knots in the workplace and public schools."

Although the CROWN Act was recognized in California and followed by many other states, I personally feel we should all do our job to support this movement to pass the law on a federal level so that this discrimination against hair can be dismantled once and for all (see Figure 1-2).

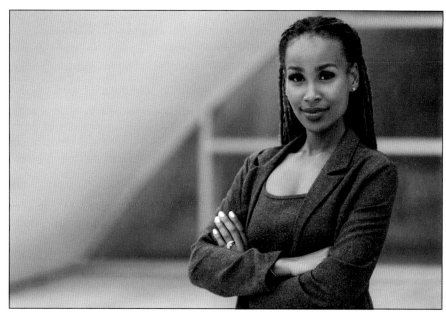

FIGURE 1-2:
Natural hair
has a place in
all workplaces.

Understanding Your Own Natural Hair History

Because this country has exhibited so much discrimination towards natural and textured hair throughout its history, people can harbor generational trauma around their hair. I talk more about this in Chapter 11. As a hair stylist, I've seen it all. Children who can't sit through hours of washing or braiding because their guardians are too rough for their tender heads. Grown adults who still flinch when it comes to certain tools because they experienced so much pain when they were younger. People of all ages constantly feeling shame or pressure to change their hair in some way that doesn't feel quite right or acceptable to them.

Many of my adult clients struggle with the fact that they were raised being told that their natural hair was not *good hair.* This could mean people told them in words. Or maybe their parents made girls get their hair straightened to "look better" to society. I have multiple clients who have clear memories of getting their hair straightened by using a hot comb every week for church so that it would look "presentable" — as though their natural hair wasn't.

In these ways, many Black and Afro-Latina women have hair-related trauma stemming from their childhood, which unconsciously taught them to hate something about their hair. This unconscious negativity can make you feel less than, and you don't even realize it.

And then those girls grow up and pass on the same hair trauma or prejudices to their own children. I remember one of my clients saying she caught herself commenting on her daughter's edges, wanting them to lay down as flat and straight as possible. For what? For some outside beauty standard that's based on the idea that what you have isn't good enough? It was a moment of awareness for my client, and she's working through it to heal so that she can better herself and her child.

Don't get me wrong; I don't hate straight hair. I love all hair types. I love helping people achieve straight hair in healthy and successful ways if that's what they want. (I give you some tips and tricks for straightening your hair in Chapters 8 and 9 of this book.) But I take issue with the fact that, so often, straight hair is deemed beautiful, but curly and natural hair isn't. Newsflash: It's all beautiful! And I'm here to help you embrace whatever style you want (see Figure 1-3).

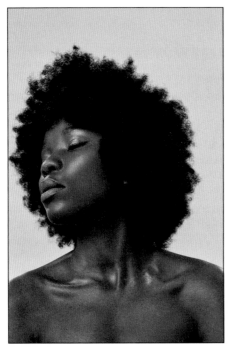

FIGURE 1-3:
Wear your afro (or whatever style you want) with pride!

© Svitlana/Adobe Stock

Getting Comfortable with Your Natural Hair

If you're just starting to transition away from a relaxer or another chemical process to grow your hair out into its natural state, congratulations! I know changes can sometimes be tricky, but I'm here to help you through it. Whether you're going to get *the big chop* (cutting all the processed hair off to start fresh, which you can read more about in Chapter 3), or simply stop using relaxers and let your strands gradually grow out, I'm here to support you through all the in-between stages while you get to where you're going.

You may find it exciting to see what emerges while you let your locs do their own thing. I go into detail in Chapter 3, but here are a few tips to get started now. You can make it a great experience by

>> Giving yourself grace and patience to trust the process: Some days will be more challenging than others, but it's a learning process.

>> Spending quality time with your hair every day: Try new products and tools to see what your hair responds to the best.

>> Taking note of the hairstyles that other people are wearing: What do you like? What makes you feel happy? Again, not everything looks the same on every person or works the same way, but you can use this time to try anything you want.

>> Accessorizing: Try out different scarves, turbans, headbands, or clips.

>> Joining groups online or in real life where you can celebrate natural hair, as well as trade hair care tips and tricks

TIP

If you need a big chop, or you simply want some professional insight and ideas, book an appointment for a consultation and/or cut with a professional hairstylist. We can provide you with a huge asset and support while you grow out your hair and discover more about your unique strands. If you need a little guidance on selecting a stylist, check out Chapter 6.

Learning the vocabulary

The language of natural and curly hair evolves every day. New styles, trends, and techniques emerge all the time, and so does how we talk about natural and curly hair. You may already know and use a bunch of these terms, but if you're just starting out and need to get up to speed on the basics, check out this quick starter vocabulary list:

- » **Big chop:** Cutting your hair very short to remove any processed hair and start fresh to grow out your natural hair.

- » **Co-wash:** When you use conditioner instead of shampoo to wash your hair.

- » **Curl pattern:** The natural shape of your hair strands.

- » **Elasticity:** Your hair's ability to return to its natural shape after you manipulate it, such as pulling, stretching, or heating it.

- » **Morning routine:** What you do to your hair every morning after you wake up to get ready for the day. You might spend every morning moisturizing or hydrating, co-washing, and/or styling. See Chapter 5 for more on getting your routine set.

- » **Naturalista:** Someone who's proud of their natural hair. They thrive on keeping it in its natural state without straightening, perming, or using chemicals or excessive heat.

- » **Nighttime routine:** Similar to your morning routine, except you get your hair ready for bed by massaging your scalp, moisturizing, setting, and covering it with a scarf. You can find more on that in Chapter 5, as well.

- » **Porosity:** How well your hair can absorb and retain moisture. Turn to Chapter 2 for how you can test your hair's porosity at home.

- » **Slip:** Lubricating products, such as conditioners, that make moving combs or fingers through your hair much easier and without friction.

- » **Transitioning:** When you stop applying relaxer to your strands and start growing out your natural hair, gradually trimming off the processed ends of your hair.

- » **Twist out:** Unlike braids, for a twist out, you twist two sections of hair together, rather than a braid's three. When you take twists down, the resulting twist out creates either a loose wavy pattern or tighter curls, depending on the number and size of the twists. You can choose from many variations of twist outs. Visit Chapter 9 for more.

- » **Wash-and-go:** When you style your hair using only your hands or wet brush and product after you wash it and let it air dry. Visit Chapter 9 for more on wash-and-go's.

- » **Wash day:** The day you wash your hair. For natural hair, wash day comes around about every seven to ten days. I cover all the ins and outs of making the most of wash day in Chapter 4.

Characterizing hair types

Hair type is the actual curl pattern that you see when you look at your hair. Types go from 1 to 4. The lower the number, the looser the curl pattern. The higher the number, the tighter the curl pattern. Also, each number is paired with a letter that describes the width of your hair. In this book, I talk about Types 2c to 4c.

The reason we talk about hair types and textures so much is because every type and texture (*hair texture* is how your hair feels when you touch it, such as coarse, thick, fine) needs slightly different hair care and styling to feel and look its best. As a stylist, I know what someone who has 3c hair needs to help their curls come alive and how their needs are different from someone who has 4c hair. The hair care profession has made everything nuanced and specific because we've figured out so much over time. Determining your (or your loved one's) hair type can help you source the right products, tools, and techniques for your personal strands.

To figure out your hair type, flip to Chapter 3.

And now, a word. Or maybe several.

I recognize that some people don't feel comfortable with this system because it puts the least-textured hair first on the list and the most-textured hair at the end of the list. But you can choose to start your healing right here. If this hair typing system bothers you, you can simply not use it and not pay it any attention. For me, the system makes sense, and provides direction and organization for hair care, so I'll leave it at that.

When it comes down to it, the hair typing system is all perspective. And if you don't like it, I encourage you to try not to let others determine your thoughts and opinions. Take control over what you want for your hair and life. That's what true healing means.

Putting some thought into your style

When it comes to styling your natural and curly hair, I want to encourage you to really take time to think, observe, and sit with what you want. Your hairstyle is about you, and you alone. Do what makes you happy.

TIP

If you don't know where to start in choosing a new style, do what I do sometimes when I'm working on a new design for a client or upcoming photo shoot. Go out and look around at what others are doing:

>> Go to the bookstore or newsstand, and look at hair magazines to see what's looking fresh.

>> Google the latest hair trends.

>> Check out social media and see what your favorite influencers are doing.

>> Refer to Chapters 9 and 10 in this book for hair styling ideas.

All of these methods can give you great ways to find inspiration and ideas for your own personal style.

Also, really stop and consider how others impact you. If "I woke up like this" is your theme song and daily mantra, do whatever you want to, haters or not. But if you know a weird look, shady side eye, or whisper will bother you, this is the time to think through that and choose something that won't make you feel small. Instead, do what makes you feel comfortable. Your hairstyle should make you feel proud, self-assured, and free no matter where you are (see Figure 1-4).

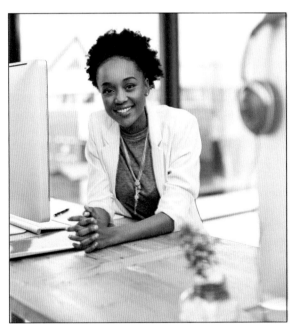

FIGURE 1-4:
A quick and easy workplace style.

© Getty Images/John Wiley & Sons, Inc.

In addition to getting in tune with what your heart wants, also consider certain logistics and practicalities, such as how much time and effort you want to spend on your hair. If you have a lot of time or don't mind a commitment to daily upkeep, go for that higher maintenance style. But if you're pressed for time in the mornings or don't have the resources for weekly salon visits, keep it on the simple side. You might also want to ponder what your local climate is like. Is it humid and hot? Dry and cold? Make sure to take that into consideration when choosing a style and the care that goes with it. Visit Chapter 6 for more on how the environment can impact your hair.

TIP

Just remember: The world is your oyster. Everyone finds figuring out new things a little hard at first, but that doesn't mean you're not up for the challenge. The more you practice creating a specific style, the easier it becomes. I applaud you for trying new things and embracing your hair in all its glory.

Keeping your hair in tip-top shape

All beautiful and healthy hair starts with the right care and maintenance. Everyone's hair is unique, so you have to experiment to find a routine that's perfect for you. What works for your friend or cousin, or even your sister, may not work for you, but all great hair care routines include a few basic steps:

>> **Wash day:** The day you wash your hair, and it typically takes hours. You need to set aside a full day usually to give proper attention to your locs. I run through this wash-day routine in detail in Chapter 4.

>> **Morning and nighttime routine:** I cover these routines in more detail in Chapter 5, but here's the bottom line: You typically need a daily routine that's split up between the morning and evening. In the morning, you style and protect your hair from the elements. At night, you need to keep your strands protected from sleeping and prime them for the next day.

>> **Protective styling:** You can use many styles to protect your hair from constant touching and the climate to keep it healthy.

Considering the best tools and products

All great hair care and styling requires the right tools and products. But with so many brands out there, how do you know what to get? It can take some time to figure out what your (or your child's) hair specifically needs. On top of that, you may find it tricky to determine which products and tools truly work. Companies make all kinds of claims to get you to buy their products, but how can you tell which ones are legit?

In this book, I devote two full chapters to this topic: Chapters 7 and 8. If you need product recommendations and reviews, feel free to skip straight there now.

I know it can seem like you have to acquire a lot of tools and products at first, especially if you're new to the curly or natural game, but just start with a few tools. Then add more along the way. Just go slowly and try things out. Some tools and products won't feel right or do what you want. So get rid of them (or give them to someone else to try). When you find something that makes your hair feel and look how you want, keep it.

You can also ask around to your friends and family members to see what they like. You don't get a guarantee that what works for them will work for you, but it at least gives you a good way to find things to try. Just keep an open mind and don't get discouraged.

Today's retail stores are more fully stocked than ever with multiple products and tools for natural and curly hair — plus, the Internet gives you a never-ending treasure trove of options.

If you need somewhere to start, here's my list of basic tools that you should have in your hair care and styling collection:

>> **Brushes:** You need one to detangle and one to dry. If you want one that does both, you can look into paddle brushes, but they don't necessarily work well for all hair types and texture.

>> **Wide-tooth comb:** Perfect for detangling and separating your hair.

>> **Fine-tooth comb:** Use this comb to create sleek hairstyles and remove scalp buildup on wash days.

>> **Rat tail comb:** Helps you style. Use it to part and section your hair like a pro.

>> **Hair pick:** Especially important for big, voluminous styles, such as afros.

>> **Hair ties:** Use silicone or cloth-covered scrunchies for when you want to wear your hair up.

>> **Satin or silk bonnets, scarves, and pillowcases:** While you sleep, these materials reduce friction and help preserve your style longer.

WARNING

You might want to try other tools, as well, such as hair dryers, curling irons, flat irons, and hot combs. Because they all involve heat, you need to be a little more cautious when you use them. I go into great detail in Chapter 8 about how to use these tools safely and when to go to a professional.

As for products, those are even more personal, and finding the right ones can take more trial and error than finding the right tools. And you can feel so overwhelmed when you look at all the different bottles, jars, and formulations.

REMEMBER Here's a guiding principle to live by when choosing hair products: Water is the most important ingredient of all. All of your products should have water (sometimes listed as *aqua*) as the first or second ingredient.

Here's a rundown of basic products to have in your collection:

- **Shampoo:** Use a clarifying shampoo to deeply clean your hair, as well as a moisturizing shampoo to moisturize it.

- **Conditioner:** Use conditioner that you rinse out after shampooing, as well as detangling (or leave-in) conditioner that you can use to comb out tangles and keep your hair moisturized. You can also use detangling or leave-in conditioner to co-wash your hair on non-wash days.

- **Edge control:** This gel-like product helps you keep flyaways down around the hairline.

- **Oils:** Use oil to keep your scalp and hair healthy and moisturized. You can find all sorts of different oils that do different things, so take your time to figure out what works the best for you. You need to experiment, but I walk you through some ideas, and a lot more info about products in general, in Chapter 7.

REMEMBER People who have natural or curly hair shouldn't wash their hair every day because it can dry out your curls. It's different for everyone, but I recommend washing once every seven to ten days.

If you want guidance on how and when to use all of these products, turn to Chapter 4, where I talk all about wash day in detail.

Styling your crown and glory

Okay, this is the super fun part. The part where anything goes. Because curly and natural hair is incredibly versatile, if you can dream it, you can do it (or, you can hire someone to do it for you).

Whether you want braids, twists, a mohawk, an afro, extensions, or wigs, it's all possible. Yes, some hair textures and types are more cut out for different styles than others, but really, you have no limits. Your hair is your crown and glory. Your true expression of self. Your celebration of your heart and what you want to say to the world.

And you can change it as often as you like.

Styling isn't just about looking good, though. You can use low-maintenance protective hairstyles for times when you need to give your locs a reprieve from constant wear and tear.

REMEMBER

Using protective styles periodically can help you keep your hair healthy and happy, as long as you don't leave them in too long.

To find the step-by-step of all your favorite styles — protective and otherwise — head to Chapter 9.

If you're a guardian of a child who has natural and curly hair, and you need a quick crash course on how to style their hair, turn to Chapter 12.

Reshaping the Natural Hair Narrative

Throughout my eight years as the hairstylist for former First Lady of the United States Michelle Obama, I got to see different types of beauty from around the world, and I witnessed firsthand how her presence in the White House gave other women of color permission to feel beautiful and helped reshape how a nation and the world see beauty. I watched little girls, little boys, and even grown adults take her in: The complexion of her skin, her powerful stature, and the always-changing hairstyle. She provided the representation that everyone needed to see to enhance their perspective on beauty.

She was in a position of power and exposure that no other person had in that moment. And her very presence in the White House challenged the beauty standards that don't serve us as a community. And I feel her presence in the White House smashed traditional beauty standards, and we continue to grow from there.

That kind of energy changes a world. And with this book, I hope to carry that energy on. You, me, and all the different kinds of beautiful people out there are better than what some arbitrary beauty standard says. We're bigger than ourselves when we hold each other up. And we're more powerful — beyond unstoppable — when we embrace our natural beauty, from root to tip.

IN THIS CHAPTER

» Exploring the basic anatomy
of hair

» Keeping your scalp healthy

» Determining your hair's porosity
and elasticity

» Getting a grasp on your hair's
natural growth cycle

Chapter **2**

The Biology of Hair

I f you picked up this book, I assume you're in some way connected to or belong to the sister- and brotherhood of curly hair. No other beauty is quite like curly or natural hair in all its glory. Rejoice, my brethren — you're one of the lucky ones! Not everyone is blessed with such tresses.

But if you haven't found the joy of the curl yet, you're not alone. Maybe you've fought with your curls or your child's curls for years by straightening them, covering them with a hat or weaves and extensions, pulling them back in tight ponytails, or wearing braids for long periods of time. However, this chapter is all about uncovering what your hair is in its raw, natural state. I've always felt like most people don't get the chance to dive super deep into biology and structure of their hair. We learn all about it in cosmetology school, but this knowledge is for everyone. The more you know about your own hair in its natural state, the more you can care for it and keep it healthy. This chapter can help you make your hair the star it was born to be — or help your child look and feel their best.

I'm here to help. Together, we're going to free the curl! Celebrate all natural hair! You can find the secrets to your best hair day ever in this chapter.

In this chapter, I go over the basics of what makes curly hair curly. Here, you can get to know the structure of hair, how it grows, and what it's made of. You can skip this chapter if you don't need or want the background, but I recommend sticking around. After all, knowledge is power! This info determines what kind of care and products your hair needs in order to thrive.

Getting to know the ins and outs of what is actually on your head and body can give you a greater appreciation for your tresses. And before you know it, you're going to be a natural and curly hair expert, showing off your best 'do at all times.

Getting Down to the Root of the Matter: Hair Structure

Hair is an appendage of the skin. Its main function is to insulate your body from the cold and the heat, and to help protect your head from physical trauma or injury. But of course, hair is also a great accessory for self-expression. Many people consider their hair to be their crown and glory: *Crown* represents the majestic beauty and power within our hair; *glory* represent a sense of pride, admiration, and respect.

The structural work of art known as the hair fiber helps to determine its *physical effects,* meaning what it looks and feels like outwardly. Texture, shine, strength, moisture retention, volume, and the frequency of growth all come from the structural elements of your hair. Everyone is born with the hair their have. You can't fight biology, even though a lot of techniques and products might promise us otherwise. In the end, figuring out your personal hair biology and structure allows you to embrace it fully and know what it needs to look its best.

Time for a basic hair anatomy lesson. A strand of hair is made up of two parts: the hair shaft and hair root. The *shaft* is the structure above the surface of the skin. It's the part you see, touch, and manipulate. The *root* is the structure beneath the surface of your skin where hair growth starts.

Just talking about the hair shaft

Knowledge is power. You can really enhance your hair care regimen by knowing the structure of the hair shaft. From this foundation, you build your hair care and styling routines.

REMEMBER

If you know your hair shaft, you know how your hair reacts to the environment, hair products, and whatever else it may encounter. It's vital information to retain on your hair journey.

The hair shaft can consist of two or three layers (see Figure 2-1):

» Cuticle (outer layer)

» Cortex (middle layer)

» Medulla (inner layer; mainly in thick hair strands)

The *cuticle* is the thin outer layer of the hair shaft. It offers the first line of defense for the *cortex* (the middle layer). The cuticle protects and seals moisture in the hair. It consists of flat keratin cells formed around the shaft, similar to the shingles on a roof. When the cuticle is intact and has balanced porosity, the hair stays healthy.

The cortex is about 90 percent of the weight of the hair shaft, which makes it the thickest layer. It consists of melanin pigmentation. Melanin gives hair its color. Most importantly, the cortex contains fibers that give hair its length, strength and resilience, and moisture content.

Finally, the *medulla* is the innermost layer of the hair shaft, typically found in thick strands of hair. It's hollow and may not exist in thinner textures. It adds to your hair's thickness and serves no real purpose.

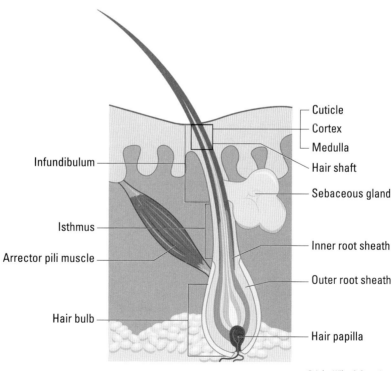

FIGURE 2-1:
The anatomy of a strand of hair and hair-root components.

© John Wiley & Sons, Inc.

Getting to the hair root

Everything beneath the surface of your scalp is the hair root. A lot of different parts make up the root as shown in Figure 2-1:

>> Hair bulb (lower segment)

>> Isthmus (middle segment)

>> Infundibulum (upper segment)

TECHNICAL STUFF

Of all the parts of a strand of hair, I'm most fascinated by the follicle because your hair follicle produces your hair shaft when it grows out from under the epidermis. At the very base of the hair follicle, you find the hair bulb. The *hair bulb* is the structure supported by active growing cells. These cells produce hair strands.

At the base of the hair bulb, you can find a structure called a *hair papilla,* a group of cells that provides oxygen and nutrients from the bloodstream, giving nourishment to the hair bulb so that it can form new hair.

A *sebaceous gland* lives right next to each hair follicle in the hair root. The most important gland for hair care, it produces and secretes the natural oils that lubricate the hair.

The structure of the cells within the hair follicle is either round, curved, or oval (see Figure 2-2). The shape of the follicle determines the type/texture of hair. Genetic attributes of the hair determine the follicle's shape.

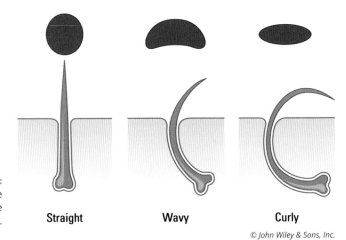

FIGURE 2-2:
The hair follicle determines the hair texture.

Straight   **Wavy**   **Curly**

© John Wiley & Sons, Inc.

If the follicle is round, the hair grows straight and generally creates straight hair shafts (so the hair you see is straight). If the follicle is curved, the hair grows back and forth, generally creating wavy or slightly curly hair. When the follicle is an oval, the hair growth generally forms curly, coily, wiry, and kinky hair shafts.

REMEMBER

With curly hair types, the bends and curves make it difficult for your natural sebum to travel down the entire hair shaft. So, you need to develop a hair care regimen that keeps your curly hair strong and moisturized. Jump over to Chapter 7 if you need help selecting a product.

Checking Out What's on Your Head

Prepare to get real comfy and cozy with your (or someone else's) luscious locs. It's time for you to commune with your coif — but don't expect it to happen overnight. Although you've had your hair with you all your life, really getting to know it is a journey, especially if you've recently transitioned from chemically straightened to natural hair (or are planning to). Your hair is more complex than it might look at first glance. It's best to be patient with yourself and take the time to get to know your hair.

First step? Appreciate your hair. Touch it. Let your fingers sink in. I'm not trying to be corny here, but if you haven't given your hair (or your child's hair) undivided attention lately, I'm giving you permission to literally embrace that curly or natural hair.

For starters, your hair not only protects your skin and stops dust particles from entering your nose, eyes, and ears, but it also provides you with one of the first representations of self-expression.

I believe hair is a language — if it's not healthy, it has no voice. Your hair is the first thing someone "hears" before you even speak. It says a lot about your personality without you having to utter a word. Your hair can express whether you're conservative, edgy, or creative. It gives insight into whether you're fun and daring, or whether you like to play it safe. Whichever way you do it, how you choose to wear your hair helps illustrate your personal story. The story starts with your scalp.

Examining your scalp

When you understand the importance of a healthy scalp (as shown in Figure 2-3), you can take charge of your hair's health, right where it starts. Of course, you need to take care of your hair itself to keep it growing healthy and strong, but you also need to take care of your scalp.

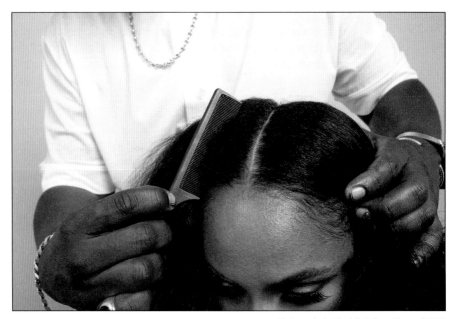

FIGURE 2-3:
Check your scalp periodically to ensure that it's healthy.

REMEMBER

The health of your hair is a direct reflection of the health of your scalp.

Keeping your scalp healthy and clean allows you to create the best environment for hair growth. An unhealthy scalp can lead to several scalp conditions, potentially resulting in dullness, overall loss of shine and luster, a rough texture, and (in the worst situations) breakage and thinning. Two of the most common conditions that affect your scalp are

» **Eczema:** *Atopic dermatitis* is a condition that makes your skin red and itchy, with occasional dryness or flakes. Children commonly have eczema, but it can occur at any age. It can be long-lasting, and usually the trigger is caused by a combination of immune system activation, genetics, environmental triggers, stress, or allergies.

» **Dandruff:** Also called *seborrheic dermatitis*, dandruff can also cause red and itchy skin, like eczema. Dandruff differs from eczema in that it causes the skin specifically on the scalp to flake in a very substantial, noticeable way. The causes of dandruff can vary from oiliness and buildup of dry skin to hormonal changes, stress, hair styling, weather, pollution, and even just simply changing your shampoo.

If you suspect you're dealing with either of these conditions, you can typically treat them with over-the-counter shampoos and treatments. The ingredients list may include

>> **Zinc:** Supports normal immune function

>> **Tar:** Reduces inflammation, redness, itching, and swelling

>> **Salicylic acid:** Softens keratin and loosens dry patches of skin

>> **Ketoconazole:** An antifungal, particularly good for bacterial infections

>> **Selenium sulfide:** An active ingredient in most dandruff shampoos, it treats inflammation

TAKING CARE OF YOUR SCALP

You can create a scalp care regimen to help prevent scalp conditions and promote overall scalp health. Here are my tips for what to include:

- **Drink plenty of water and try to maintain a healthy diet.** Foods such as fish, eggs, and leafy greens are especially good for hair and scalp health.

- **Get a scalp massage.** Massaging your scalp helps blood circulate to your hair follicles, which encourages hair growth. A massage also helps remove dead skin cells from the scalp.

- **Use a clarifying shampoo.** A good clarifying shampoo can thoroughly cleanse the hair and scalp without drying them out, and it can also balance the moisture in both hair and scalp. For help with selecting the right clarifying shampoo for you, head to Chapter 7.

- **Use an apple cider vinegar (ACV) rinse.** If you have an oily scalp or buildup of product, debris, dirt, or dead skin cells, ACV can help by balancing hair and scalp pH. By reducing the pH of your scalp, ACV flattens and closes the hair cuticle, which makes your hair smoother and less difficult to detangle, shinier, and much less frizzy. This treatment leaves your hair more moisturized, and it prevents breakage. Visit Chapter 4 for an easy DIY recipe and instructions for using an ACV rinse.

- **Exfoliate your scalp.** Scalp exfoliation makes room for fresh, new skin and for hair follicles to grow healthy, strong hair by removing dead skin cells on the scalp. This creates a well-groomed surface for the hair follicle to push up through freely. You can find several great scalp exfoliating scrubs available to purchase online or at retail stores. Exfoliate every month and a half to two months before you shampoo to make your hair shiny, keep your product buildup at bay, and improve the impact of your hair products.

If the OTC (over-the-counter) route doesn't work for you, go straight to a dermatologist. After they examine your scalp and diagnose you properly, they can prescribe you medicated shampoos and treatments to help control the condition.

Determining your hair's porosity

To really get to know your hair, you need to identify its porosity.

Basically, *porosity* is a measurement of how your hair retains and absorbs moisture. Experts typically break down porosity into three classifications (see Figure 2-4):

>> **Low porosity hair:** Fairly healthy, but does not absorb or retain enough water. Its cuticle layer (remember, it's the outside part of the hair shaft) is tighter, making it difficult for this hair to absorb product. To help low porosity hair absorb product, you can use heat or steam treatments (see Chapter 4 for more on steam treatments).

>> **Normal/medium porosity hair:** Ideal and much easier to maintain than low porosity hair. Having normal porosity hair gives you a great indication that your hair is healthy. The cuticle layer is relatively loose, and moisture can easily penetrate the hair. The more moisture that penetrates the hair, the healthier it is.

>> **High porosity hair:** Has a raised and overly *porous* (open) cuticle. Because high porosity hair is very open, it tends to be excessively dry, frizzy, and easy to snap. When your hair is highly porous, it can take in water but not retain it because of damage to the cuticle layer of the hair shaft. You get this kind of damage usually from coloring, heat styling, or too much tension from braids or ponytails.

FIGURE 2-4:
The cuticle of the hair strand determines its porosity.

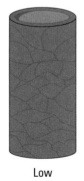 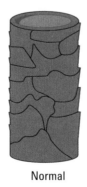 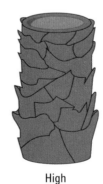

Low   Normal   High

© John Wiley & Sons, Inc.

You can test your hair's porosity at home in one of two simple ways. You perform both tests on clean and dry hair before you apply any product:

>> **Take a strand of hair from your comb or brush and drop it into a clear glass of water.** If the strand floats at the top, you have low porosity. If the strand slowly sinks towards the bottom, you have normal porosity. And if it sinks to the bottom immediately, you have high porosity.

>> **Run a couple strands of hair between your index finger and thumb, going from the ends towards the scalp.** If the strands feel smooth, you probably have low to normal porosity. But if the strands feel rough, the cuticle layer may be too loose and open, indicating high porosity.

After you know your porosity, you know whether your curls need moisture, whether they're damaged, or whether they're healthy. Porosity also gives you a better understanding of the best conditioners and treatments to use, as well as the appropriate method to layer your styling products. Visit Chapter 7 for more info on choosing products based on your hair's porosity.

TIP

Although natural porosity is genetic, different factors can impact and change it. Getting a lot of exposure to heat, chemicals, or pollution can make your hair highly porous. If you want to lower your porosity, try applying protein treatments (more on that in Chapter 4) or deep conditioning or apple cider vinegar rinses (see Chapter 7 for how-to's on those techniques).

Determining your hair's elasticity

In addition to porosity, identifying the elasticity of your hair can tell you volumes. The *elasticity* of your hair is an estimate of how much it can stretch and still return to its original shape. The elasticity helps determine your hair's overall strength.

There are three levels of elasticity:

>> Balanced

>> Low

>> High

When you have a good (balanced) level of elasticity, your hair can stretch up to 50 percent of its length without breaking when pulled; after it's released, it can return to its original length and shape. When you have balanced hair elasticity, you have defined and strong curls.

Low elasticity leads to delicate strands that you need to handle more carefully. This unhealthy or damaged hair can stretch to around only 20 percent or less of its length before breaking, and it may not return to its original length and shape afterwards.

High elasticity is usually an indication that the hair has been over-manipulated or over-processed with products or chemicals. This hair has stretched too much and appears mushy, lifeless, and sheds easily.

So how do you figure out your hair elasticity? You guessed it — test it! Testing for elasticity lets you know if your hair is moisturized well, if it lacks protein, or if it's weak.

You can test your hair's elasticity pretty easily by following these steps:

1. **Pick a strand of hair from different areas of your head.**

   Choose hairs from the front, back, crown, and sides.

2. **Spray the strands with water.**

3. **Over a white background (so that you can see it clearly), grip both ends of a hair between your thumbs and index fingers.**

   Pull the hair slowly and firmly (but not too aggressively). Try to maintain the same pressure in both hands. Then pay close attention to what happens:

   - If your hair barely stretches and breaks instantly when you pull it, your elasticity is very low. Your hair is weak because it's losing moisture faster than it should.

   - If your hair stretches and goes back to its original length and shape, the elasticity is balanced, and it's safe to say that your hair regimen has a good balance of moisture and protein.

   - If you get a lot of stretch before the strand breaks, you have high elasticity hair that needs protein. Add protein treatments to your hair care regimen. See Chapter 4 for more on that.

4. **Repeat Step 3 for each hair strand you want to evaluate.**

TIP

You may find that different strands from different areas of your head test differently. Depending on the results of each section, you may want to adjust your hair care regimen to help build elasticity in the specific areas that have the least amount of stretch.

Identifying hair breakage versus shedding

I already know — no matter what I say — that you hate seeing all that hair in your brushes and combs, on the bathroom floor, or accumulating in the drain.

But honestly, hair shedding is 100 percent a natural part of your hair growth cycle, and it happens every single day. So don't stress about it at all. You have no reason to worry about natural shedding.

You can lose anywhere from 50 to 100 strands per day, depending on the phase of growth (see my breakdown of the phases of hair growth in the following section). Sometimes, you may notice more than 50 to 100 strands if you skip brushing and combing your hair daily. You may also notice more hair shedding if you wear braids or a *sew-in* (a weave that's sewn into your braided or cornrowed hair). When you have your hair in these styles, the hairs that want to shed naturally day by day collect until you take down your sew-in or undo the braids.

You can easily identify shed hair. It's the full length of the hair strand, and the hair bulb (which I talk about in the section "Getting to the hair root," earlier in this chapter) may still be attached to the end.

Breakage, on the other hand, is a different story. Pay close attention if you notice small, little wisps of hair falling to the floor while you comb or brush. That's definitely a sign of breakage — book a consultation with a professional so they can determine the cause and come up with a breakage battle plan.

Several different things can cause breakage, including neglected split ends and snapped strands. You can cause breakage with excessive tugging and pulling, heat damage, and even intense dryness. Take breakage as a sign that your hair shaft is experiencing some type of abrasion (which basically means it's weakened or thinned). Abrasion can occur from heat damage, wear and tear, or too much tension from tugging and pulling.

TIP

Avoid breakage due to neglected split ends by scheduling to get your ends trimmed every eight to ten weeks if you heat style or once every three months if you avoid heat styling.

Grasping and Maximizing Growth Cycles

Have you ever noticed that sometimes, it seems like your hair never sheds, while other times, you shed hair like crazy? That's because your hair grows in three phases as illustrated in Figure 2-5:

>> Anagen (growth)

>> Catagen (transition)

>> Telogen (rest)

TECHNICAL STUFF

Each strand of hair grows at its own pace, so not all hairs are going through the same phase of growth at the same time. If all the strands went through the same phases at the same time, all of your hair would fall out at once.

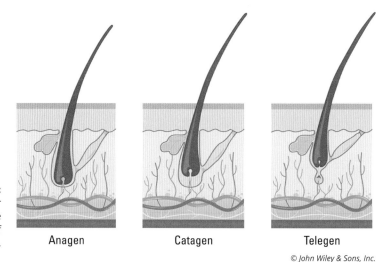

FIGURE 2-5:
The hair growth cycle consists of three stages.

Anagen   Catagen   Telegen

© John Wiley & Sons, Inc.

Anagen

The stages of hair growth begin with the *anagen phase,* in which hair actually grows. It's the longest phase, and it typically lasts about three to five years. (Although, for some people, a single hair could continue growing for seven or more years.) During this phase, new follicle cells grow at the hair bulb, generating new hair. (I talk about what makes up a hair strand in the section "Getting Down to the Root of the Matter: Hair Structure," earlier in this chapter.) At any given time, 70 to 90 percent of hair is in this phase of growth. The longer your hair remains in the anagen phase, the longer it grows.

The average growth of healthy hair is approximately ¼ inch (0.6 cm) to ½ inch (1.3 cm) a month. Most women's scalp hair grows faster than that of men. Scalp hair generally grows fuller and faster between the ages of 15 and 30, but slows down after the age of 40 to 50.

So the next time one of your friends wonders why they can't grow hair to save their life, while they watch your hair gain 2 inches seemingly overnight, tell them, "Sorry, my hair is probably just more anagen than yours." And then savagely toss your hair. No, but really, you can comfort them by telling them it's not about what they are or aren't doing, it's just the luck of the genetic draw.

Catagen

Catagen is the transition phase. It starts when the anagen phase ends and tends to last about ten days or so. After years of growing, the hair cells stop reproducing. The hair follicle begins to lose moisture, shrinks, and separates from the hair papilla (remember, the cells at the very bottom of the hair bulb that supply blood and nutrients to the follicle). Yet the follicle remains in place during its final days of growing. About 1 to 5 percent of your hair is at this stage at any particular time. The catagen phase occurs while another new strand of hair begins to grow at the root. This phase lasts from one to two weeks.

Telogen

The telogen phase typically lasts around three to four months. An estimated 10 to 15 percent of your scalp hairs are in this phase at any point in time. Hairs don't grow during the telogen phase.

During this phase, new hairs start to form in the follicles that released hairs during the catagen phase. The follicle eventually grows out of the skin to create a new shaft. When new hairs sprout to the surface of the scalp, they push out old strands or remains of strands. The new hair strand enters the anagen phase, which begins a new cycle.

So now that you know a little about the different phases of hair growth, you can tune into and understand a bit more about your own hair growth patterns.

REMEMBER

At any given time, all of your hair strands are growing, transitioning, resting, or shedding. If you ever notice that you're losing more hair than seems typical for the hair cycle or you personally, talk to your doctor to figure out whether the hair loss is related to a medical problem.

Chapter **3**

Getting to Know Your Hair

G etting to know your (or your child's) hair might sound like a simple or trite idea, but the more you know about it, the better you can care for it. And I don't mean just in general; your hair has characteristics that are specific and unique to you. In Chapter 2, I discuss basic hair anatomy, but in this chapter, I help you figure out your personal "hair ID," as I call it. In other words, no two heads of hair are the same. Your hair has its own identity that is comprised of your type, texture, density, and other characteristics. The exact combination of these characteristics is specific to you, and each characteristic thrives best with different care. I'm here to help you get to know and love yours so you can create the hair care regimen that's best for you.

But before I go any further, I want to say this: *All* hair is good hair. The type or the texture doesn't matter; having good hair means having healthy hair. Period! Never label your hair bad based on ethnicity or appearance. Regardless of your hair's genetic origins or whether it's straight, wavy, curly or coily, the only bad hair is unhealthy hair. All hair can become unhealthy, whether from damage, lack of knowledge about products and styling techniques for your particular hair type, or not having a maintenance routine appropriate to your hair type. The key to keeping your hair healthy is knowing as much as possible about it.

In this chapter, I outline the (sometimes controversial) numbering system we hairstylists use for curly hair. I give you detailed lists and information for all hair types and varying textures in that system. I also go into how to transition away from chemically treated hair to your natural hair. And finally, I set you up with tips and insights to help you appreciate your unique head of hair and hopefully point you in the "Wright" direction towards a beautiful healthy hair journey.

Defining Your Hair Texture and Type

You inherit your hair type and texture, which are determined by your genetics. Although most people use the terms texture and type interchangeably, they're two different things. As a professional, I'm here to lay out those differences so that you can empower yourself with this next-level insight. Magazine celebrity beauty secrets have got nothing on this.

Your hair *texture* is the circumference (or thickness) of each individual strand (meaning the shaft of the hair; flip back to Chapter 2 for discussion of the parts that make up each strand of hair). Your hair *type* simply refers to your hair's curl pattern that comes as a result of the shape of your hair follicle. It's the most basic formation and characteristic of the hair strand.

So why do you need to identify your hair texture and type? The short answer is, not all curly and natural hair is the same.

In the world of natural and curly hair, Andre Walker, stylist for Oprah Winfrey, created a numbered classification system that helps you to hone in on how to care for your hair in the best way (more on this in later chapters). Some say that we no longer need a system that lists, categorizes, or classifies natural and curly hair types by numbers or letters. The naysayers think this system is divisive and can possibly diminish the uniqueness of Black hair textures because the numbering hierarchy places straight hair at the beginning and textured at the end. I understand why people feel badly about that, but to me, it's a waste of energy.

Systems simplify ideas and help people gain a desired result. I've been a professional hairstylist for over 30 years, and I've been fortunate enough to see curly hair types from people all over the world — including some who don't identify as Black. I believe that categorizing hair textures not only makes it easier to identify them, but also celebrates our differences, empowering those who have all kinds of natural and curly hair textures — curl-power!

If you want to determine your exact type and texture, don't worry; I'm here to help!

Feeling out your texture

The *Milady Standard Cosmetology*, 13th Edition textbook, an industry standard among cosmologists, divides hair texture into three types: fine, medium/normal, and coarse.

Fine

Fine hair is the most fragile texture. It feels soft and silky to the touch, but you can easily damage it. Believe it or not, if you have fine hair, you may have a larger number of hair strands than people who have thicker hair strands. But because your strands have less structure, they can't easily hold a style or volume. They often fall flat or look limp and thin.

WARNING

Fine hair is normally oiler than other hair textures because they have more hair per square centimeter and each hair has a sebaceous oil gland, which produces more oil. Plus, you can weigh it down by using heavy products, making the hair look stringy.

Structurally, fine hair contains only two layers:

» **Cuticle:** The outermost part of the hair shaft

» **Cortex:** The thickest layer of the hair shaft and the layer that contains the hair pigment

To see an illustration of your hair's anatomy in its entirety, flip back to Chapter 2.

Medium

Medium hair feels silky to the touch, but it's stronger and not as susceptible to breakage as fine hair. Medium hair can hold styles fairly well. It's fuller and covers the scalp, but you still don't want to do any excessive heat styling because it can damage your curls. If you have medium-texture hair, you can use moderate heat a few times a year without worrying about doing damage. (For more on heat styling, visit Chapter 8.)

Structurally, medium hair contains two to three layers — the cuticle and the cortex (which I talk about in the preceding section), and sometimes the *medulla* (the innermost layer of the hair shaft).

REMEMBER

A lot of people call medium hair *normal* because it's the most common hair texture. So I mention that term in case you hear it in your travels. But all hair is normal, and that's just pure facts.

Coarse

Coarse hair is strong and can feel both silky and rough to the touch, depending on its level of moisture. It has a lot of volume because each strand of hair has the largest and widest circumference of any other texture. Because of how large the strand is, coarse hair has the tendency to need extra hydration; it may lose moisture more quickly than the other hair textures. If you don't manage coarse hair properly, it can become dry and brittle, making it vulnerable to breakage. Coarse hair takes longer to dry, holds styles well, and can tolerate higher amounts of heat.

Structurally, coarse hair has the most protein of the three textures, and it contains all three layers: the cuticle, cortex and medulla (discussed in the preceding sections).

TIP

But don't go too crazy with heat styling if you have coarse hair. Too much heat can rob your hair of moisture. Aim to heat style only about four times a year. You can go up to six if you're keeping your coarse hair in good shape.

Finding your type

Hair types are separated into four categories, and then into three subcategories: Types 1 through 4, and then A, B, or C for each number. For each type (and subtype), I describe the characteristics so that you can pick the type that seems most like yours. This book mainly focuses on hair types 2c to 4c, which are shown in Figure 3-1.

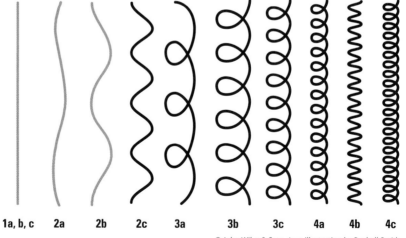

FIGURE 3-1:
Hair typing
chart.   1a, b, c   2a   2b   2c   3a   3b   3c   4a   4b   4c

Curls come in all shapes and sizes, and you might even have more than one hair type on your head, so don't be surprised if you recognize yourself in more than one description. However, most people typically have a dominant hair type, so if your multitextured hair is confusing to you, just focus on the most dominant one (the one you have the most of).

Type 2

Type 2 falls somewhere between straight and curly hair. It's normally flat at the root of the hair follicle. Most people think of Type 2 hair as wavy, and it ranges from gently tousled textures to S–shape defined waves. You can have fine to coarse Type 2 hair, but it's typically fine. Here are the three kinds of Type 2 hair:

>> **2a:** Loose, stretched S-shaped waves

>> **2b:** More distinct S-shaped waves

>> **2c:** The most defined S-shaped waves that can form loose ringlets and spirals (see Figure 3-2)

Of the three Type 2 subcategories, 2c is the closest to curly hair types, so I want to give you a detailed description of 2c.

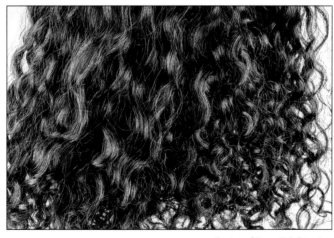

FIGURE 3-2: Loose ringlets and spirals are the main features of Type 2c hair.

Courtesy of KnappyHair Extensions

Type 2c hair can require a lot of maintenance. Here are a few good habits to help keep your tresses happy and healthy:

>> **Use a clarifying and volumizing shampoo on wash day.** Depending on how oily and weighed down your hair gets, you might want to shampoo twice a week (for the complete guide on wash day, visit Chapter 4).

>> **Use a lightweight conditioner, and focus your application of it towards the ends of your hair.** Heavy conditioners can cause your hair to fall flat and limp. Alternatively, you can go with a light leave-in conditioner. (Need help finding the right product? Jump ahead to Chapter 7.)

>> **Try products that add moisture and volume/thickness.** Volumizing and thickening products help thicken your fine hair without weighing it down.

>> **Air-dry your hair until it's about 75 percent dry before you style it.** Wet hair is very fragile and can easily break while you pull and stretch it. If you use a diffuser, be sure to dry your hair with your head upside down to create volume at the roots.

>> **Schedule regular hair trims.** Get a trim every six to nine weeks. Because fine hair is so fragile, it tends to split more often. Regular trims prevent your split ends from traveling up the hair shaft.

>> **Try to limit heat styling.** Fine hair is vulnerable to breakage. Because heat styling can accelerate breakage, I don't advise it.

>> **Don't overuse your styling product.** Apply your favorite products sparingly. With fine hair, a little goes a long way.

>> **Choose mid- to shoulder-length hair cuts that use textured layers.** Long, fine hair can stretch your curls out, causing your hair to appear much thinner than it actually is. The ends are the oldest part of your strands, so when you leave them on, they are less full. Keeping a shorter hair cut keeps it looking fuller because the hair closest to the root is the newest and thickest.

>> **Apply protein treatments monthly.** Most hair types can benefit from protein treatments. It makes the hair stronger and adds a layer of protection for fragile hair. Hop over to Chapter 4 for the 411 on these treatments.

Type 3

Type 3 hair is S-shaped curly hair that ranges from springy, tight corkscrew curls to loose, bouncy curls with more volume at the roots (see Figure 3-3). Type 3 hair has some shine, but if you don't give it enough hydration, these curls can have issues with frizz and *curl definition* (which is how well and clearly you can see the shape and pattern of each curl individually). Type 3 hair can be fine to coarse, but it's typically medium-textured. Here are the three kinds of Type 3 hair:

>> **3a:** Big, loose, well-defined spiral curls

>> **3b:** Bouncy, tighter ringlets and spiral-shaped curls that have a lot of volume

>> **3c:** Even tighter, corkscrew curls on the verge of Type 4 curls

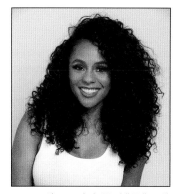
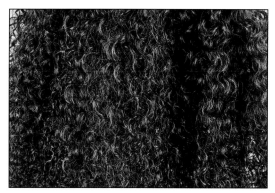

Photography by Wardell Malloy with crowdMGMT

Courtesy of KnappyHair Extensions

Type 3c hair can experience *shrinkage*, where your hair strands appear shorter when they're wet.

Type 3 hair is less fragile than Type 2, but you still need to nurture it properly. Here are some good habits to keep them curls poppin':

>> **Detangle every wash day.** Type 3 hair can be prone to matting if you don't detangle it before shampooing. Need me to walk you through that process? Skip ahead to Chapter 4.

>> **Use traditional shampoos and conditioners once a week.** Type 3 hair tends to need more styling products than Type 2, so shampooing weekly prevents buildup. Also, your curls yearn for moisture. Conditioning weekly keeps your moisture balance consistent.

>> **Schedule regular hair trims.** Get a trim every six to nine weeks.

>> **Switch to deep conditioners or a hair mask every other wash day.** You can apply these products in addition to or instead of your traditional conditioner. Deep conditioners and hair masks penetrate deeper into your hair's cuticle and help prevent frizz, enhance curl definition, hydrate the hair, and restore your curls.

>> **Add slip with leave-in conditioners.** Leave-in conditioners give your curls *slip* (that means they reduce friction and allow curls to move freely). They also add moisture, making your hair more manageable and easier to detangle.

>> **Use oils or oil-based styling products.** When it comes to moisturizing natural hair, water is the holy grail. Oils and oil-based products help seal and trap moisture in your hair.

If you need help selecting the right products for your hair, visit Chapter 7.

Type 4

Type 4 hair has S-shaped or zigzag curls that are very tightly coiled (see Figure 3-4). These curls are normally described as coily and kinky. Type 4c hair can shrink more than 50 percent of its actual length when wet. Because we're all uniquely made, 4c hair can have fine to coarse texture. But the most common 4c texture is coarse and may have noticeable curls with less definition. Here are the three kinds of Type 4 hair:

>> **4a:** Tightly coiled S-shaped curls that begin at the scalp and continue throughout the shaft to the ends

>> **4b:** More tightly curled than 4a hair, with more of a zigzag curl pattern

>> **4c:** Super tight zigzag curl patterns with less curl definition

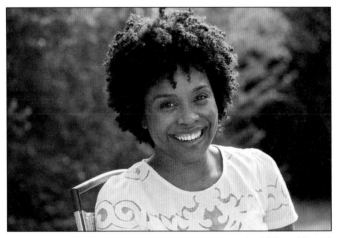

© digitalskillet1/Adobe Stock

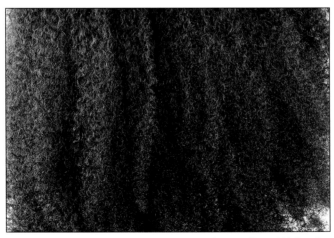

FIGURE 3-4:
Type 4 hair is tightly coiled.

Courtesy of KnappyHair Extensions

Good habits for Type 4 hair are similar to the habits for Type 3 hair, but Type 4 comes with a few tweaks and extra tips:

>> **Detangle first,** as always. Detangling is important for all wash day routines. Make sure you detangle your hair to keep it healthy and unmatted.

>> **Weekly, first detangling your hair, then use a moisturizing shampoo or shampoos formulated for coarse hair.** Some shampoos for coarse hair may be listed as sulfate-free. (You can find more on detangling in Chapter 4.)

>> **Every wash day, use a deep conditioner or hair mask.** You can use this deep conditioner either with or instead of your regular conditioner.

>> **Incorporate steam treatments biweekly with your conditioner, deep conditioner, or hair mask.** Steam treatments can moisturize and hydrate all types, but it really helps coarse hair get the extra hydration that it needs. Chapter 4 offers information on steam treatments.

>> **Limit using alcohol-based products.** Although these products help tame your hair, they can strip hair of moisture. Instead of alcohol-based products, use oils and creams that help seal moisturize and hydrate.

>> **Use a detangling brush while your hair is wet.** Detangling brushes help remove knots, which keeps your hair from breaking and becoming damaged.

>> **Schedule regular trims.** Coarse hair can be prone to split ends because of its tendency to be dry. I recommend getting regular trims every eight to ten weeks.

>> **Try co-washing biweekly.** Co-washing may or may not work for you, but it doesn't hurt to give it a try. (I go into more detail on co-washing in Chapter 4.)

>> **Choose products for anti-shrinkage and enhance curl elongation.** Chapter 7 has more on these products.

TIP

Sleep with a silk or satin head covering or pillowcase, which protect all hair types. These fabrics reduce friction, frizz, flyaways, and breakage, so you can more easily maintain your curls. See Chapter 5 for more information on nighttime routines.

Getting Clear on Density

Get to know your hair's density. Now, a lot of people confuse hair density, type, and texture, which I totally understand. I talk about texture and type in the section "Defining Your Hair Texture and Type," earlier in this chapter. But I'm going to lay out the density details for you right here and now.

Density is the amount of hair strands per square inch of your scalp, so how close your strands grow next to each other. A person can have low, medium, or high density. The average person has nearly 2,200 strands of hair per square inch, which roughly adds up to about 100,000 strands on your head.

TIP

Someone who has fine hair can also have high-density hair. They grow a lot of fine hair per square inch on their head. On the other hand, someone can also have thick or coarse hair and low density, which means you have thick strands, but you don't grow as many strands per square inch. You can find just about any combination of texture and density, but you get my point.

If you want to measure your hair's density, here's how you can do at home yourself using the parting (or scalp) test. When your hair is dry and in its natural state, look in the mirror and use a rat tail comb to part your hair down the middle. Here's how to identify which hair density you have:

>> **Low density:** Your part seems wide, and your scalp is very visible.

>> **High density:** Your part is very narrow, and you can barely see your scalp.

>> **Medium density:** Your part size and scalp visibility fall in between low and high density.

Your hair density is mostly based on genetics, but stress, health conditions, hormonal changes, and (more commonly) age can all affect it. While we age, our scalps shrink, and we lose follicles, which directly changes our hair density.

REMEMBER

Knowing your hair density doesn't necessarily determine how you should take care of your hair or what products to use (that's more for hair type and texture). Rather, knowing your hair density can make a big difference in choosing your perfect style or haircut.

Here are my quick picks for best styles and cuts based on density:

>> **Low density hair:** Choose short to mid-length haircuts.

   Avoid going past the top of your bra line. Select cuts that have strong lines that create weight, paired with soft layers around the crown that add fullness.

>> **Medium density hair:** Your selections for haircuts and styles are endless — have at it!

>> **High density hair:** Choose cuts that involve graduated mid-length to long layers.

These styles help remove weight. Your stylist can thin your hair by using thinning shears to help remove weight, create more texture, and help make dense hair more manageable.

USING AI TO FIND YOUR HAIR ID

As an educator, I love being able to give you the nuts and bolts of the science behind your hair so you can understand your hair fully, but I know trying to identify your hair type and texture can sometimes feel overwhelming or confusing when you are navigating different descriptions, charts, and tests.

Well, I have an absolutely *amazing* solution for you that helps take all the challenge away. It's called Myavana, and it is positively *revolutionizing* the natural and curly hair world with its groundbreaking technology! It seriously blew me away the first time I learned about it.

If you need help figuring out your hair type and texture and which products are the best for you, Myavana (short for "my hair nirvana") has you covered. Myavana is a beauty technology company that has a consumer app by the same name. (I recommend that you head right over to wherever you download apps to get it immediately!) You simply upload a photo of your hair, the app analyzes it using proprietary science, and creates a hair profile for you.

Myavana helps you discover the current state of your hair, which it calls your "Hair ID." Your Hair ID combines your true hair texture, type, and — here's what really sets it apart — your hair's condition (your hair's porosity, elasticity, density, and overall health).

If you have a combination of hair type and texture that a photo analysis cannot analyze, you can order their Hair Strand Analysis Kit, similar to 23&me, for a more comprehensive analysis and healthy hair care plan containing recommended products, regimens, and a local stylist in a digital hair profile. They have created a whole ecosystem of consumers, product manufacturers, salons, retailers, and distributors to lead the digital transformation of the hair industry.

You can get a comprehensive hair analysis, Unique Hair ID, and digital healthy hair care plan with the Myavana Hair Strand Analysis Kit available at www.Myavana.com/pages/journey-to-hair-nirvana?utm_source=johnnywright.

At the time of writing this book, I entered a partnership with Myavana, which may entail a fee to promote the service and app.

TIP

I absolutely love giving you information that helps you get to know and love your unique head of hair. But if you're still finding it difficult to determine your hair type, texture, or density, schedule a consultation with a *trichologist* (a specialist in the hair and scalp) or licensed hairstylist (look for their certificate posted at their salon). A detailed consultation can help you figure it all out and lead you to a great relationship with your beautiful curls.

Making the Decision to Go Natural

We all know that change is inevitable, but we also know that deciding to change isn't easy. Transitioning from relaxed to natural hair is a complex move to make. It demands patience, consistency, and a great deal of commitment. Whether you're thinking about the big chop or just growing out your relaxer, when you decide to go natural, you have to commit to a completely different way of styling and caring for your hair.

Ask yourself three main questions when you're trying decide whether to go natural:

» **Do I have the patience for this?** Patience is essential. Just like anything in life, you have to be patient to see progress. Although it'll take some time, I'm certain that with the help of this book, you can end up with great results.

» **Am I ready for a big change?** Most people are emotionally connected to their hair. People associate it with wealth, status, and even royalty. Your hair helps you illustrate your personal story and your personality. We use the way we style our hair to communicate identity and self-expression. Don't make the decision to go natural just to follow a trend. Make this decision based on how you want to show up in this world and take back the power of how the world defines beauty.

» **Do I have the time to care for natural hair?** Honestly, natural hair requires time and maintenance. Oftentimes, you might want to try natural hair if you see a celebrity or influencer who has natural hair or you come across a picture online or in a magazine. But you don't see the work it takes to achieve those styles. Deciding to go natural means adapting to new products and styling techniques that might take extra time and practice, so go in with realistic expectations and a good attitude. You may find it challenging at first, but after you get the hang of it, it becomes second nature.

Transitioning to natural hair

Most people who relax their hair have been relaxing it since childhood. And even if you have a few botched attempts to go natural under your belt, you might have yet to really stop relaxing your hair long enough to know exactly what your natural hair has to offer.

You need an understanding of how your hair grows. In particular, how fast it grows. Hair growth varies from person to person, but on average, hair grows about a half-inch a month. That puts most people right at six inches per year. In order for you to know what your natural hair texture has to offer, you should let your hair grow out 6 to 8 inches, depending on your type and texture.

REMEMBER

In other words, transitioning your relaxer out enough to see your natural hair can take about a year or more.

Here are some tips to help you grow out your relaxed hair:

>> **Avoid excessive heat styling.** Excessive heat styling compromises your curls and creates an uneven curl pattern and breakage.

>> **Try wet sets with flexi-rods or perm rods.** Flexible curling rods (also known as *flexi-rods*) are small individual cylinders around which you wrap your hair to curl it. After shampooing and conditioning — while your hair is wet — comb out and split your hair into small enough sections for the size of rod you select. Then place a rod at the end of each section and tightly roll the hair into it. Flexi-rods and perm rod sets create beautiful curls and voluminous hair without direct heat (in other words, using a hooded hair dryer on medium to high heat will not damage your hair). See Figures 3-5 and 3-6.

>> **Steam treat often.** Many people find that while their natural hair pushes through, the relaxed hair tends to break. This breakage happens because the natural texture is strong and creates a line of demarcation where the relaxed hair stops and the natural hair starts, causing the relaxed hair to become fragile and break because the difference between the two is so stark. It's not the same for everyone — it's particularly true for the more textured hair types, like 4c. Steam treatments paired with your favorite conditioner can help soften that line of demarcation and promote less breakage.

>> **Trim your hair when needed.** Trimming every six to ten weeks, depending on your hair type, helps speed up the process. I know it doesn't make sense, but trust me on this. Trimming regularly helps to prevent split ends from traveling up the hair shaft, which can cause damage to your new curls. Regular trimming also keeps your fragile strands from breaking by removing weight.

>> **Detangle gently and carefully.** Because the line of demarcation makes the hair weaker, take your time while detangling. Use your fingers rather than combs and brushes to detangle. Gently rake your fingers through sections of your hair to remove knots and tangles. See Chapter 4 for more on that. In general, finger detangling helps you minimize breakage because you have more control over it.

>> **Select products that keep your hair moisturized.** Start experimenting with new products. Avoid drying ingredients. All hair, first and foremost, needs moisture — but transitioning hair particularly needs it. While your curls grow in, it becomes more difficult for your natural oils to travel down the hair shaft. Definitely start using new products that keep your hair hydrated. Flip over to Chapter 7 if you need help selecting some new products to try.

CHAPTER 3 **Getting to Know Your Hair** 47

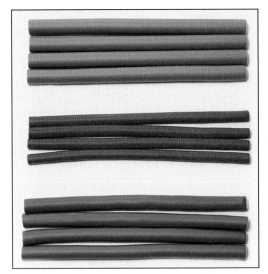

FIGURE 3-5:
You can use
flexi-rods for a
fabulous look.

Photography by Wardell Malloy with crowdMGMT

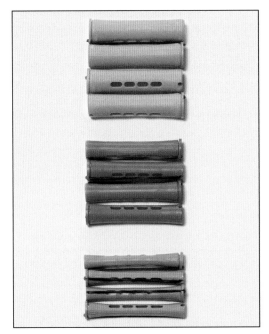

FIGURE 3-6:
Perm rod
sets are a
great tool to
have on hand
when you're
growing out
your relaxed
hair.

Photography by Wardell Malloy with crowdMGMT

>> **Remember to add protein.** Hair is made up of 80 to 90 percent of a protein called keratin, which gives hair its strength. Make sure you use a product that includes plenty of keratin along with your moisturizer. Otherwise, hair can

actually become weak and nonresponsive to styling and hold. See Chapter 4 for more on protein treatments.

>> **Incorporate protective styles into your styling routine.** Part of the challenge of growing your hair out is that you don't want to touch or manipulate it too much. But if done properly, protective styles can help you minimize manipulation and assist in your transition journey. Although I don't recommend it often, all protective styles (such as braids and sew-ins) can minimize friction and breakage by giving your hair a moment where nothing (and no one) touches it. In Chapter 9, I go over everything about protective styles.

>> **Don't stress over shedding.** Shedding is natural, and transitioning hair sheds a lot. Outside of the usual 50 to 100 strands that the average person sheds daily, you may see a tad more while transitioning. Don't trip — it's totally normal, so you don't need to stress.

Choosing to do the big chop

Ahhh, the dreadful big chop. I know, just the thought of it makes you cringe and bite your nails. You don't have to take such a drastic step. You can cut a little at a time working up to it over a few days or weeks, or you can choose to be dramatic and cut it all off at one time. It's totally up to you.

Going natural isn't a new thing, but recently, the hair world has experienced a surge of women who are cutting their relaxed or chemically treated hair off (known as *the big chop*) as the beginning of a new journey towards embracing their natural hair. Whether a little a time or all at once, some women just want to cut it all off and start over in hopes that it grows back healthier (see Figure 3-7).

What comes next if you do the big chop? Here's what you can look forward to:

>> **Enjoy a sassy, bold new haircut.** You definitely turn some heads and may even open up a whole new world of attention.

>> **Cut down your prep time.** For obvious reasons, you can cut your glamming-up time in half. Just getting up and going without having to put too much effort into your hair can be a game-changer.

>> **Embark on a whole new hair journey.** Now, you can get to know your natural hair and its versatility. You can play with new products and different ways to manipulate your hair texture.

Many people just go for it and reach for the nearest pair of shears or clippers to chop it all off. But for the best results, and to find out all your options, consult with a professional hairstylist or barber.

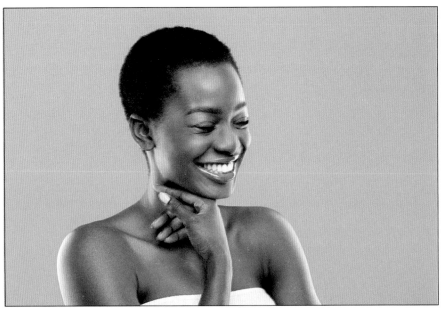

FIGURE 3-7:
The big chop.

Navigating the in-between stage

REMEMBER

Growing out your natural hair can take up to 2 years. A majority of that time, your hair lives in that awkward, in-between stage — the stage where you start to question why you decided to go natural in the first place. You consider chopping it back off with every glance you take in the mirror. Honestly, you just can't think short term. Keep the bigger picture in mind, and remember that patience and commitment play a huge role. In the end, you can proudly say you saw it all the way through.

People can find the in-between stage so stressful and challenging that I once saw a "The In-Between Stage for Natural Hair" online support group. (Hey, it may still be out there if you need it.) The struggle is real, and you are not alone.

If you don't have the time or money to book with a stylist, you can go to Part 4 of this book for suggestions. You can also find countless DIY options online, including on YouTube. You can wear a wash-and-go, twists, braids, or sew-ins, which I go into more in Chapter 9. You can also buy accessories to help you spruce up your look. The most important thing is to keep your growing hair healthy and be patient, and I guarantee you'll be happy after you get to your desired length.

2

Maintaining Your Natural and Curly Hair

Fine-tune your wash day by following step-by-step instructions for detangling, washing, conditioning, and treating your hair.

Keep your hair happy and healthy by creating a great daily routine.

Protect and preserve your locs by moisturizing, using head coverings, and getting regular trims.

IN THIS CHAPTER

» **Establishing a schedule for wash day**

» **Detangling do's and don'ts**

» **Caring for your scalp**

» **Shampooing, conditioning, and co-washing secrets**

» **Treating your hair with a little extra oomph**

» **Drying your hair without drying out your hair**

Chapter **4**

Fresh and Clean: Wash Day

The most basic way to take care of your hair is to wash it, but you need to know a lot about how to handle your hair when it's wet and — quite frankly — the most vulnerable.

If you're like most people, you probably have a love-hate relationship with your beautiful kinks, coils, and curls: especially on wash day. Each week, you procrastinate as much as possible by co-washing or using your favorite style-refresher products to go as long as you can between washes. Am I right?

I know it's not that you don't want clean hair. It's all the sectioning, detangling, pre-washing (if needed), shampooing and conditioning, setting, drying, and finally styling. It's exhausting. Trust me, I get it.

Here's the trick, though: Creating a routine and sticking to it can make wash day less of a chore and more of a delightful experience. Wash days should be experimental and fun — and hopefully something to look forward to.

If you've lost the joy in your wash day (or never had it), I'm here to help. In this chapter, I go over how often to wash your hair, how and when to detangle, the joys of co-washing, and (most importantly) how to properly shampoo and condition, along with other tips you can use for wash day. This chapter shows you how to play around with new products and give your hair some love through proper care!

Setting Your Wash-Day Schedule

Of course, your wash-day schedule all depends on your specific hair type and texture, but as a professional, I generally recommend that folks wash their hair at least once per week. You can go longer between washes, but don't go any longer than two weeks. If you have finer hair or extra buildup, you can try washing your hair twice a week. (You can refer to the section "Figuring out how often to shampoo," later in this chapter, for guidance.)

Choose whatever schedule works best for your needs. Just keep in mind that to have a successful wash day, you need to do all the steps I outline in this chapter — and do them in order! Make sure you have time for detangling, shampooing, conditioning, and any drying or additional styling at the end. So choose a day in which you have at least a couple of free hours. You can't rush good hair care!

TIP

If you have especially coarse, dry, or damaged hair, you can use another technique called *co-washing*, where you use conditioner in place of shampoo. I go into more detail about this process in the section "Co-Washing," later in this chapter.

Ow! Detangling Your Hair

The first step of any wash day is detangling. For some people, detangling their hair can be the most tedious and time-consuming process of a wash day. But fear not! I've got you covered from root to tip.

The detangling process is different from person to person, but here's some guidance that can help you minimize excessive snagging and breakage.

First and foremost, set aside enough time. Detangling can take anywhere from 15 to 40 minutes. I know, I know. You might be tempted to skip this step, but don't. If you wash your hair without thoroughly combing and detangling your hair first, you can make your tangles worse by matting them when you add shampoo and excessive water during the wash step (which you can read all about in the section "'Pooing Like a Pro," later in this chapter).

I don't recommend detangling dry hair because it's less flexible than wet, and you can end up damaging your hair's cuticle. However, if you choose to detangle your hair dry, do not rush! Go very slowly! It's important to be extra gentle to avoid snapping strands or damaging that cuticle. And if you have extra thick or coarse hair, you're going to have to dig deep and be extra patient.

When you're preparing to detangle your hair, you can make the process go more smoothly if you have the right tools on hand. Get yourself:

» A rat tail comb

» A wide-tooth comb

» Your favorite detangling product to add some *slip* (lubrication that reduces friction, making it easier to move combs or fingers through your hair) to your hair strands

» A few clips or ties (see Chapter 8 if you need more info about and a little help selecting these tools)

Now that you have the right tools at the ready, follow these steps to detangle your hair:

1. **Use a rat tail comb to section your hair into at least four to eight sections, depending on how thick and dense your hair is.**

   You can use hair clips, hair ties, or loose *plaits* (braids) to keep the sections separate. Working in small sections makes your hair more manageable and ensures that you're thoroughly removing all the knots. Pre-sectioning can help give you more control over your mane and set you up to properly detangle. I've been a professional hairstylist for over 20 years, and still to this day, one of my most useful styling practices is pre-sectioning.

2. **Add a softening agent to your hair, such as a detangling or leave-in conditioner.**

   Keeping your curls hydrated while detangling creates important slippage. Chapter 7 has more information on selecting detangling or leave-in conditioners.

3. **If your hair is extra tangled, try finger detangling first.**

   After sectioning and moistening your hair, start at the ends of one section. Slowly separate the hair in that section with your hands, removing shed hair, tangles, and knots while you go. Take your time. If you rush and try to yank or pull, you could damage or break your hair further.

   Also, if your hair isn't very tangled at all, you may be able to get away with just finger detangling and don't need to continue on to the rest of these steps!

4. **Comb the hair out with a wide-tooth comb (see Figure 4-1) or a detangling brush, one section at a time.**

Start at the ends and work out any knots while you travel up to the roots. This process prevents unnecessary tugging and pulling at the roots, which causes more damage.

Use a plastic cap to cover the sections that you haven't detangled yet. This cap helps stop your hair from drying up.

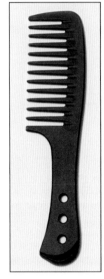

FIGURE 4-1:
Use a wide-tooth comb to detangle your tresses.

Photography by Wardell Malloy with crowdMGMT

With curly hair, you need to create as little friction as possible, so detangle your hair only on wash day, as long as you can keep it in good condition between washes. In other words, detangle only once every one or two weeks. You may find the need to finger detangle a little more often between wash days if you're styling has interrupted your curls, or you forgot to sleep in your bonnet, or something like that.

TIP

Sleeping in a silk or satin head covering or on silk or satin pillowcases can help minimize friction and maintain your curls between wash days.

Taking Special Care of Your Scalp

Healthy hair begins with a healthy scalp, and a healthy scalp is a clean and moisturized scalp. Washing and conditioning your hair regularly — at least once a week — is great for basic maintenance, but if you use a lot of product (which most naturalistas do), you should first clean and nourish your scalp with apple cider vinegar, tea tree oil, or peppermint oil (or any combination). *Note:* You use each of these scalp treatments at different times and in different ways.

Here are a few tips on using these treatments during your wash day:

>> **Apple cider vinegar (ACV):** After you shampoo and before you condition your hair, combine 2 tablespoons of apple cider vinegar with 5 tablespoons of water. Using an applicator bottle, distribute the mixture evenly across the scalp, massaging it in for a bit. Leave the mixture on for 5 minutes, then rinse it out. ACV balances and soothes the scalp, removes buildup, and heals dry and itchy scalps.

>> **Tea tree oil:** Avoid applying pure tea tree oil to your scalp. Dilute about 2 tablespoons of tea tree oil with 1¼ cup of coconut oil, aloe vera, or even apple cider vinegar. You can also add tea tree oil to your favorite shampoo. When mixing your own tea tree oil solution, start with a concentration of 5 percent. This concentration translates to 5 milliliters (mL) of tea tree oil per 100 mL of the carrier substance. Apply the mixture directly to your scalp, leave it on for about 5 minutes, then rinse it out. Tea tree oil is antibacterial, anti-inflammatory, is a great dandruff treatment, and improves overall scalp health.

>> **Peppermint oil:** Before you shampoo, apply the peppermint oil directly to your scalp, massage for about 2 to 3 minutes, and then let sit for 15 minutes. Don't worry, you're supposed to feel a tingling sensation. After 15 minutes, you can shampoo and condition. The main benefit of peppermint oil is that it increases blood circulation on the scalp, which helps your hair grow.

WARNING

Just to be safe, always do a patch test before using any new product to ensure you're not allergic to it. Apply a couple of drops of vinegar or oil to a small patch of your skin and monitor that patch for any irritation for at least 24 hours. After you get the all clear, you can add the vinegar or oil to your wash day.

'Pooing Like a Pro

REMEMBER

You must remove all tangles before shampooing to prevent matting (a giant clump of tangles that is hard or impossible to remove with a comb or brush alone), so if you haven't detangled yet, back up and visit the section "Ow! Detangling Your Hair," earlier in this chapter.

Figuring out how often to shampoo

The main purpose of any shampoo is to remove dirt and oil residue from your hair and scalp. Shampoos help you cleanse your hair of its natural *sebum* (the oil your sebaceous glands produce to keep your hair and skin naturally moisturized and protected from bacteria), remove residue and buildup from styling products, and prepare your hair to fully accept the moisture you deposit on it during conditioning (which I talk about in the section "Conditioning Your Curls, Kinks, and Coils," later in this chapter).

I recommend people who have curly or natural hair not shampoo their hair too often, although you don't want to go too long between washes, either. Extended periods of not washing your hair can cause odor, buildup, and dandruff on your scalp, and you can even hinder your hair's ability to grow. When residue from products or sebum builds up, blocking your hair follicles, your hair can't push out and grow. The residue also starts to weigh your hair down and can lead to breakage.

Everyone's level of sebum and product buildup is different depending on things such as fitness routines (or how often you sweat, in general), environment, product use, and how much oil we produce naturally. Some people need to shampoo more often than others. Do what works best for your hair. Throughout this journey, you will have to do a lot of trial and error to find your best shampoo routine. Start with little bits at first, then add more if needed.

The ins and outs of shampooing twice

If you want A-list locks, you need an A-list wash setup. I have a secret tip to start you out that can automatically elevate your hair game. On wash day, I always suggest shampooing twice, using two different shampoos, before applying conditioners, treatments, or hair masks. The first time, use a clarifying shampoo. The second time, use a moisturizing shampoo, which helps soften your hair and replenishes its moisture. (If you need help picking shampoos, flip to Chapter 7.)

Starting with a clarifying shampoo strips your hair of all its residue and gets it squeaky clean because of its strong, effective ingredients that fully remove dirt, oil, and hair products. A nice clean scalp and roots ensure your hair can grow freely.

WARNING

However, because a clarifying shampoo is so good at stripping your hair, in some situations, it can make your hair dry or brittle; that's why I recommend following your first clarifying shampoo with a gentler moisturizing shampoo. If you don't like that squeaky clean feeling for your hair, you can use a gentle moisturizing shampoo for both washes.

With this insider information, you're now ready to start your shampoo adventure. Follow these steps:

1. **After detangling, make sure you have your two shampoos.**

   See the section, "Ow! Detangling Your Hair," earlier in this chapter, for more on getting those tangles out.

2. **Thoroughly wet your hair, using lukewarm water.**

   Using lukewarm water while you shampoo your hair opens up the cuticle of the hair shaft and the pores in your scalp, making them ready to accept the moisture you add while shampooing and conditioning.

3. **After you fully saturate your hair, pour about a quarter size amount of shampoo into the palm of your hand.**

   Use whichever shampoo you prefer.

4. **Distribute the shampoo at your hairline, then all over your scalp.**

REMEMBER

   Massage the shampoo on your scalp with the tips of your fingers (not your nails). Your grip should be firm enough to help lift residue off the scalp but not so hard that it becomes uncomfortable. Massaging your scalp also stimulates blood circulation, which is essential for hair growth.

5. **After you build a good shampoo lather, rake your fingers through your hair, spreading the shampoo from your scalp to the ends of your hair.**

   Raking your hair with your fingers while you shampoo helps keep your hair from tangling again. Continue massaging and raking for 2 to 3 minutes.

6. **Rinse thoroughly and repeat as you prefer.**

TIP

Depending on how dense your hair is, use more than a quarter size of shampoo for each wash, if needed.

Conditioning Your Curls, Kinks, and Coils

After you shampoo, your hair needs a conditioner to add radiance, strength, and manageability, as well as softening and closing your hair's cuticle. Conditioners are key to your wash-day routine because they counteract the drying effects of shampoos by providing hydrating agents known as *humectants* to your hair. Chapter 7 gives you more on humectants, as well as how to select rinse-out and leave-in conditioners.

Although rinse-out conditioners and leave-in conditioners both help to hydrate and moisturize your hair, they have different roles, and you use them completely differently.

Rinse-out conditioner

Rinse-out conditioners rehydrate hair and also help protect it from future damage. To use them, follow these steps:

1. **After you finish shampooing, while your hair is still wet, apply a generous amount of conditioner to your hair.**

   It's important to spread the conditioner evenly throughout your hair, making sure all your hair is well saturated with conditioner.

   To help you spread your conditioner evenly, use a detangling brush, paddle brush, or wide-tooth comb to work in the conditioner and comb out any extra tangles or knots created from shampooing.

3. **Let the conditioner stay on your hair for a period of time.**

   I'd suggest 5 to 10 minutes, but you can also follow the instructions on the conditioner's label. Just give the conditioner enough time to do its job.

   If you have time, you can cover your head with a plastic cap to trap in your body heat or sit under a dryer or steamer for added heat while you let the conditioner do its magic to your hair.

   With heat, conditioners can penetrate deeper into the hair for more effective and longer lasting results. You can find more tips and tricks about how to use heat to your hair's advantage in the section "Steam treatments," later in this chapter.

5. **Rinse your hair thoroughly.**

   Rinsing the hair with cool water will help close the cuticle and promote shine.

LOOKING AT THE LOC METHOD

If your hair feels dry to you, you can use the three-step LOC method to keep your hair fully hydrated and moisturized and your curls well-defined. LOC stands for leave-in conditioner, oil, and cream.

Although you can technically use this method whenever you would like, I recommend doing it on wash day. If you do it every day, you may find the extra product in your hair leads to build-up on your scalp.

To use this method, gather your favorite leave-in conditioner, oil, and cream. To your freshly cleaned hair, apply each product individually to your hair in order of the acronym: leave-in conditioner (L) first, then oil (O), and finally, cream (C). You can use as much or as little of each product as you want. The idea is to layer each product on top of the previous to create ultimate hydration and moisturization.

You can use the LOC method no matter what your hair type or texture is, but if you have high porosity hair, the LOC method can be especially helpful when you are combatting dryness. Also, if you have tighter curls, the LOC method works very well in helping you define your curls without weighing your hair down with product. If you have looser curls, you can still use the LOC method, but I would recommend using less product or lighter-weight products so you don't weigh your curls down.

Leave-in conditioner

Leave-in conditioners are a curl's best friend. They help to protect, hydrate, and boost your hair's texture and malleability while minimizing frizz. You can use them to add extra moisture — especially if you have some damage from heat or other styling techniques, if your hair feels drier than normal, or if you have color treated or bleached hair. You can never go wrong with more hydration.

TIP

Use a light spray or leave-in conditioner if you find that your moisture level leaves your hair feeling or looking too greasy for your liking.

Like the name suggests, leave-in conditioners are made to not be rinsed off, so you should leave them on your hair until your next wash day. The ingredients are a little different from rinse-out conditioners, so if you usually use a rinse-out conditioner, expect leave-ins to be a little lighter. Leave-ins are excellent for hydrating your hair between washes and providing that extra layer of protection.

They can also assist with detangling. Follow these steps to use a leave-in conditioner after you thoroughly rinse out the rinse-out conditioner from your hair:

1. **Towel dry your hair so that it's just damp, and then apply leave-in conditioner.**

   Be sure to follow the instructions on the label for the suggested amount of leave-in conditioner to use.

2. **Use your fingers or a wide-tooth comb to spread the conditioner evenly through your hair.**

3. **Style your hair as desired.**

   Alternatively, you can let your hair air dry.

TIP

You can also use a small amount of leave-in conditioners on dry hair between wash days. Use them whenever you feel like your hair needs a quick pick-me-up, or to refresh your style.

Co-Washing

Have extra thick, coarse, or dry hair? Co-washing may be your way to give your hair extra moisture and hydration!

Co-washing may sound like something it isn't. Co-washing doesn't involve getting a friend to wash their hair at the same time that you do. The *co* in this case is short for *conditioner. Co-washing* means that instead of shampoo, you use conditioner to "wash" your hair, hydrating it.

To co-wash your hair, follow these steps:

1. **Gently finger detangle your hair.**

2. **Fully saturate your hair with water.**

3. **Apply conditioner to your hair, also massaging it deep into your entire scalp.**

   Apply the conditioner just like you do regular shampoo.

4. **Fully rinse the conditioner out right away.**

   Spend twice as much time rinsing as you spent massaging the conditioner in. ***Note:*** Don't let the conditioner sit on your hair; just massage it in, then immediately rinse it out.

5. **Use your rinse-out conditioner again. This time, you only need to apply it to your strands, and not your scalp. Then rinse out thoroughly.**

   (For conditioner how-to's, flip back to the section "Conditioning Your Curls, Kinks, and Coils," earlier in this chapter.)

Not everyone wants or needs to co-wash, but if you do because you want to avoid shampoos or feel like your curls can benefit from the extra hydration, do it on your wash day. Just keep in mind that co-washing doesn't actually cleanse your hair. It really serves solely to deeply hydrate it with all of the conditioner's heavy moisturizing ingredients. I highly recommend alternating shampoo wash days and co-wash days because shampoo wash day cleans, but strips, and co-wash day moisturizes but doesn't clean. On one wash day, co-wash. Then the next wash day, do a regular shampoo to make sure your hair and scalp have a chance to get truly cleaned of things like

>> Sweat

>> Dead skin cells

>> Sebum

>> Hair product

>> Dirt

>> Environmental pollutants

WARNING

I don't recommend co-washing if you have fine, loose curls or wavy textured hair because the extra conditioner tends to weigh hair down.

If you need help with selecting a conditioner for co-washing, head over to Chapter 7 for more info on how to pick the right product for you.

Handy Tools: Using Your Fingers

Having a complete collection of tools to assist you with your daily routine is a dream come true for most people. But did you know there are styling techniques that you can do with your own bare hands? Let's talk about it!

Scrunching

Scrunching is a styling technique that quickly adds volume and definition to you waves and curls after you have shampooed and conditioned. To use this handy technique, you cup your hair in your hands or a microfiber towel and squeeze to help shape your waves or curls. Scrunching doesn't damage your hair and is very easy to do. This technique works best for 2c to 3c hair types. Here's a step-by-step:

1. **On freshly cleaned, conditioned, and detangled hair, apply your favorite curly hair products from roots to ends.**

   The products should moisturize, defined, and hold your curls. Go to Chapter 7 if you need help picking a great product.

2. **Separate your hair into sections for control and manageability.**

3. **Grab a handful of a section and cup the ends of your hair, gently squeezing while working upwards toward the roots.**

4. **Repeat until you've scrunched each section and have shaped your curls to your liking.**

5. **Let your curls air dry and scrunch from time to time for more curl definition while it dries.**

   Alternatively, you can scrunch with a blow dryer and diffuser attachment to dry your hair faster.

TIP

To add fullness and volume to your scrunch, diffuse your hair upside down.

Praying hands

The praying hands method helps you get the most out of your wash-and-go by giving your more days with your curls between wash days. The praying hands method is a technique for smoothing generous amounts of products throughout your hair. This helps with even product distribution and minimizes frizz. With this technique, you simply rub product on both hands, place a section of your hair between flat, praying hands and smooth product on the hair from root to ends. This method gives you smoother and a bit more elongated curls that will last longer.

You can also refresh your curls on day three or four between wash day with the praying hands method. This technique is perfect for when you want to avoid completely disturbing your curls but want to freshen them up a bit without causing more frizz. Just spray a little water on the ends, use the praying hands method to apply more product and smooth out the curls then scrunch at the ends to pop those curls back into shape.

Raking

Raking (aka rake and shake) is a technique you can use to rake products through your hair with your fingertips, somewhat mimicking a wide-tooth comb. This helps to detangle, define, and smooth curls section by section. To get started, section freshly cleaned damp hair into four to six sections. Work from the nape of the neck upwards, applying products on each section. Using your fingers, rake from roots to ends and as your fingers move closer to the ends of each section, gently shake your hand to loosen and defined your curls. The gentle shake will help your curls fall naturally. Once you've raked each section, diffuse to dry, and you're done.

WARNING

To avoid frizzing, don't manipulate your curls too much while drying.

Once your hair is completely dry, apply your favorite lightweight shine products to give your curls a more polished finish.

Shingling

Out of all the curly hair methods, shingling requires the most patience because it can take a lot of time. However, when you do it correctly, shingling works well on all curly hair types and textures. It is especially great if you struggle with a lot of shrinkage. Shingling is a wash-and-go styling technique where you apply products like leave-in conditioners, curl creams, and curl defining gels on your hair while separating, stretching, and smoothing the product onto every curl.

Again, work in small sections, and it's best to start at the nape of the neck and work your way up. Air drying is best for the shingling method but you can also use a diffuser to get it at least 50 percent dry if you don't have the time.

TIP

While shingling, keep a spray bottle handy to keep hair from drying out.

Adding Moisture: Hair Treatments

In addition to the basic wash-day methods I cover in the preceding sections, I want to go over a few other treatments. Natural hair is very diverse, and so are wash-day methods. The differences in curl sizes, how your hair reacts to damage, your individual strand thickness and overall density, shrinkage and elongation, and water retention all play a role in making everyone's hair just a little different from everyone else's (go back to Chapters 2 and 3 for a refresher on the biology of hair and individual type and texture). The following sections discuss other wash-day methods that you can use along with or instead of shampooing and conditioning. After all, you don't have to follow any rules in your personal natural hair journey. *You do you!*

Hot oil treatments

Hey curl-friend, do you even realize how much you put your hair through? From detangling, washing, styling, braiding/twisting, high and low tight ponytails, coloring, heat styling and all the constant tugging and pulling, it can all cause a lot of wear and tear on your tresses.

Hot oil treatments can definitely come to the rescue. After you detangle and before you shampoo, you can use hot oil to treat dry scalp and dandruff caused by moisture loss. You can also use it to reduce hair frizz and help prevent split ends, as well as stimulating blood flow to your scalp.

For the best results on natural hair that's dry, brittle, or damaged, use hot oil treatments ideally once a week, or at least every 2 weeks. Apply a hot oil treatment to your strands and cover your hair with a plastic cap for up to 30 minutes; then rinse thoroughly. After you start seeing improvements, you can reduce your treatment to just once a month to maintain your hair health. For help choosing the right hot oil treatment, flip to Chapter 7.

Steam treatments

In the World According to Johnny, steam treatments are the number one way to keep your curls popping and in top shape.

A steam treatment not only makes you feel like you're at the spa, but steaming is one of the best things you can do to hydrate your dry kinks, coils, curls, and waves. Steam can refresh all levels of curly hair textures to maintain curl definition and elongation.

Steaming simply involves using moist heat to help gently lift the cuticle layer of your hair, enabling your topical oils, conditioners, masks, and other product treatments to penetrate deeper. This penetration allows better absorption of moisture into the hair strands. Steaming also helps remove impurities such as product buildup, oil residue, and salt from the scalp's sweat glands.

You can steam your hair every wash day, right after you shampoo. Grab your favorite conditioner or mask, saturate your hair with it, and then clip your hair up. Sit under a hood steamer (you can get different models for your home use) for about 15 to 20 minutes, then rinse thoroughly. Trust me, your curls will thank you when they come out well-defined and hydrated!

If your hair feels extra parched, dry, or on the verge of damage or breakage, you can increase your steaming time to 20 to 30 minutes. Depending on the health of your hair, you might need to steam even longer. The key is to let your hair sit in the steam long enough for your cuticles to lift and absorb the treatment.

TIP

You can find all kinds of steamers available on the market, from professional-level tabletop or stand hood steamers to handhelds, but guess what? You can even steam without having a steamer!

If you don't own a steamer, here's an easy DIY steaming hack. The steam generated from a warm, wet towel can be just as effective as a traditional steamer.

Just follow these steps:

1. **After shampooing, saturate your hair with your favorite rinse-out conditioner or mask.**

2. **Soak an absorbent towel in water.**

   If you have a turban towel, you can use that. Turban towels are great for keeping your hair compact enough to keep it neat and fit under the dryer.

3. **Heat the towel in the microwave for 1 to 2 minutes.**

   Get the towel very warm, but not scalding.

4. **Lightly wring out the towel so that it's not dripping wet.**

5. **Wrap the towel around your head.**

   Make sure to gather up all of your hair in the towel.

6. **Leave the towel on until it is no longer hot.**

7. **Repeat Steps 2 through 6 one or two more times, then rinse your hair thoroughly.**

Protein treatments

A protein called keratin makes up a significant portion of your hair, but as your hair grows out over time, the ends lose moisture. This causes the keratin to break down (which is one of the things that leads to split ends). For healthy hair, you not only need to take care of the protein that is in your hair already, but you can add extra protein to it by doing protein treatments. Protein treatments help strengthen your hair follicles, improve elasticity, reduce breakage, and just overall make your hair look healthy!

If you have especially dry or damaged hair, or your hair has high porosity (flip back to Chapter 2 for help with identifying your porosity), protein treatments are extra important and helpful!

You can go to a salon for a professional chemical protein treatment one to four times a year, or you can do a DIY protein treatment on a monthly (or even weekly) basis. I recommend doing it at home for a more natural approach that you can apply more often.

Here's how to do your own protein treatment at home:

1. **Apply your chosen protein treatment product starting at your scalp and working your way down to the tips of your hair.**

   Use your fingers to rake or a wide-tooth comb to comb distribute the treatment evenly and thoroughly.

2. **Wrap your hair into a bun.**

3. **Cover your hair, if needed (refer to the product manufacturer's instructions).**

4. **Sit under a hood dryer on low heat for the recommended number of minutes by the manufacturer.**

5. **Remove the covering, untwist your hair, and rinse out the conditioner.**

6. **If needed, shampoo and condition according to the manufacturer's instructions.**

Drying Methods

After you cleanse and moisturize your scalp, detangle and shampoo, and condition, the final step in your wash-day wizardry involves drying your clean, moisturized hair. You can accomplish this drying feat in all sorts of ways. I encourage you to try different methods to find what works best for you. See how your hair reacts to each approach. You might be surprised — your favorite technique to do may not be your hair's favorite!

Keep in mind, you don't have to dry your hair at all. It's your hair and your life! If you prefer to just wash and go, head over to Chapter 9, where I give you all the info you need to air dry your hair.

Goodbye, cotton — hello, microfiber!

If you like to use a towel to squeeze out water from your hair to dry it, switch from cotton to microfiber. Microfiber towels are an excellent hair-care tool because they're specifically designed to create less friction and therefore less frizz! Even though you can find regular cotton towels just about everywhere, they're actually pretty terrible for your hair. Cotton towels create a lot of friction, which means more frizz. And check out this bonus of microfiber towels: They also help prevent breakage because of the *lack of friction!*

Give yourself the shirt off your back

If you don't have a microfiber towel, try a t-shirt. It's one of the best ways to dry natural hair. I'm serious! Soft, smooth t-shirts are perfect for absorbing water without the friction of a typical bath towel. The material is much better for hair.

TIP

If you're in a hurry, try plopping your hair! *Plopping* is a super easy and effective technique in which, essentially, you wrap your hair in a t-shirt while you move onto something else. By the time you finish doing that something else, the t-shirt has worked its magic! Follow these steps to start plopping:

1. **Place a clean cotton t-shirt on your bed.**

   You can also place it on your couch or another low, soft surface.

2. **Flip your head upside down and dangle your hair above the shirt.**

3. **Bring the shirt up around your hair like you're going to put the shirt over your head, but stop short.**

   Position the waist of the shirt around your head near the neck and the chest of the shirt around your hair.

4. **Flip your head back to a standing position.**

5. **Make sure that all of your hair is tucked into the shirt, and then use the sleeves to tie it off.**

6. **Let your hair stay in the shirt for as long as you need.**

   Usually, keeping your hair wrapped for about 10 to 15 minutes gets it as dry as you need it.

When you take the shirt off, you might even gasp at how amazingly dry — yet soft and flowing — your hair feels.

Using the natural air to dry your natural hair

This hair-drying method doesn't offer anything super-secret or fancy, but I do want to assure you that air drying is a totally legit and healthy way to go. It's low maintenance and great for people who don't like a long routine.

Just gently squeeze out excess moisture — as much as you can — and then go about your day. That's it! Your hair can stay damp for a bit, and you can usually apply styling products to damp hair.

Hairdryers do it faster

Let me just go on record right now: If you use a hairdryer, go for it! No shade or shame here.

Using a hairdryer on natural hair is safe, fast, and effective, if you follow these important tips for avoiding damaging your hair:

>> Apply a rich moisturizer or heat protectant to avoid drying out your hair.

>> Use a low temperature heat setting.

>> Attach a diffuser to distribute the heat more evenly over your curls to help prevent frizz.

Wash day is a big day for hair, and it's super personal. Take your time and experiment to figure out what works best for you. Don't get discouraged if it takes a little time to reach your personal perfection. Remember to be adventurous and patient while you experiment to find the best way to care for your precious curly or natural hair. You and your hair deserve it!

Chapter **5**

Your Daily Root-ine

With so much information floating around, almost everyone feels overwhelmed when they decide to go natural. You have to choose from so many products, styling tools, techniques, and accessories, the options can feel endless. Truth be told, the options *are* endless. But no matter what, you can keep your curls looking and feeling their best with the right daily routine.

Curly and natural hair needs tender love and care. Adapting to a daily routine and keeping it consistent provides that TLC. Think of it like brushing your teeth: You brush your teeth every day to keep your smile healthy. Giving attention to your strands daily definitely keeps them healthy and happy. Just like your weekly wash-day routine (which I talk about in Chapter 4), you can create a daily styling routine that works for you. After you figure out what routine works best, with a little help from this chapter, that routine just becomes a normal part of each day.

You might put together a daily routine that involves technique, products, tools, and accessories. And just because a particular product or technique works for your good curl-friend, that doesn't mean you can necessarily get the same results. Very few methods work for everyone. No one-size-fits all routine exists. So, to identify an effective daily routine, you need to get to know your hair and find out what it can tolerate. Remember, outside of the advice from a professional hairstylist, you're the expert on your hair.

Managing Your Expectations

No matter where you are in your natural and curly hair journey, this book can help you manage your expectations. If you're transitioning, change is never easy, and embarking on a natural hair journey definitely comes with challenges. If you've straightened your hair all your life, you have a huge decision to make — whether to go natural. Even if you're already rocking your natural or curly hair, make the daily investment of loving and celebrating it.

You may find that testing out new products, working with new tools, getting to know your curl pattern, and figuring out how much time you need to devote to your haircare regimen may seem quite daunting in the beginning (or at any point, really). Becoming a natural hair pro doesn't happen overnight. Despite all the books you read, videos you watch, and curly hair seminars you attend, you'll fall into some pits that you need to climb out of. But you expect some setbacks in any journey, right? Being patient with yourself is key.

You may look at your bestie's shiny, luscious, beautiful, well-defined curls and think they have it all figured out (see Figure 5-1). At the moment, maybe they do — but I can guarantee you that they had to make a daily commitment to figure it out. And I can also guarantee that comparing your curls to your bestie's curls can lead to nothing but frustration. In any natural hair journey, you need to embrace your unique head of hair and know that throughout the process of figuring out what works for your curls, you definitely have to go through some trial and error. Each day, expect to have successes and challenges.

Here's a list to help you manage daily expectations during your natural hair journey:

>> **Expect to feel excited about and enjoy the process — and get annoyed with the process at the same time (maybe all in the same day or same hour).** If you're a first timer to natural hair, it's like any new relationship. In the beginning, you love everything about them. But over time, when you both get comfortable, you start noticing things you're not so crazy about. If it's a relationship worth keeping, you hang in there and figure it out. In the beginning of your hair journey, you get so excited when you start to see your curls coming through. You find products that work and techniques that help minimize your routines. But while your hair grows, your texture can slightly change. The products you fell in love with don't work the same on your hair anymore. Be flexible and expect to switch it up from time to time.

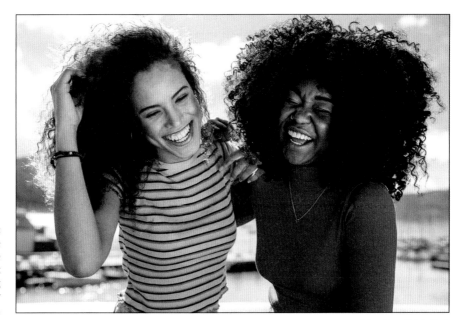

FIGURE 5-1:
Your curly bestie can give you the encouragement you need during your natural hair journey.

>> **Don't do a big chop if you're not comfortable or simply don't want to.**
I only recommend cutting it all off when the majority of your hair is damaged. But if you have healthy hair, you can successfully transition relaxed hair to natural hair over time, little by little every day. Just expect to experience more shedding than normal because of the line of demarcation between the two textures. Whatever path you choose, just focus on keeping your hair well moisturized daily.

>> **If you decide to go with the big chop, the in-between stage while it grows out can drive you crazy.** You may struggle to find styles that work and don't look matronly. You face frustration with the daily grind of looking at and trying to work with your in-between stage when growing out your curls. But good things come to those who wait.

>> **Prepare to experiment with products and routines.** Although the products I recommend in this book generally work for the majority of people with curly hair, they don't work for everyone. You face very high odds of spending and wasting a lot of money on products. I'd even say it's a guarantee. Even when you think you found the *it* product or combination of products, your hair may react to seasonal changes, and you find yourself back at the beauty supply store or surfing online. Before you know it, available space on your bathroom shelves and countertops noticeably shrinks.

>> **Make sure that you have some coins available to spend on new tools and accessories for your routine.** From detangling brushes and wide-tooth combs, to satin or silk pillowcases and bonnets, to headbands and hair ties, you can save yourself a ton of time and anxiety in the long run by loading up with the best tools and accessories. But don't worry about having to buy everything at the same time. You can add things to your daily routine gradually while you try different items.

>> **Try a protective style to keep your daily routine a little easier.** Protective styles can minimize the amount of manipulation your hair experiences on a daily basis and can really help the growing-out process. If you want to, give a protective style a try. But keep in mind that you should do your research before choosing one. Go to Chapter 9 for more on those styles.

>> **Don't assume that every style works for you.** You'll constantly be inspired by styles you see on other people, both in real life and on various forms of media. Don't assume that feeling of inspiration means that particular style will look good on you. While you experiment with your hair during your daily routine, take notes and remember the successes. Strive to find three to four go-to styles that you know look great on you and that you can easily create so that you have options during your morning routine.

>> **Expect the frizz.** No matter how much frizz-defying product you use on your curls, you still may have some frizz. Don't look at frizz as the enemy. A little frizz can add character to your style. If I give my two cents, I suggest embracing it and letting it *do what it do*.

>> **You can't always get immediate curl definition.** Using hot tools for your hair is one of the hardest habits to break. Frequently reaching for hot tools to help define your curls doesn't help your curl pattern. Avoid excessive heat styling as much as possible because too much heat can dry your hair out, change the shape of your curls, or even burn the strands or scalp. While your hair grows, you can figure out ways to manipulate curl definition without heat.

To love your natural or curly hair, you not only need to let go of harsh chemicals and excessive heat styling, you also need to connect to whatever your personal culture is, and let go of what society has prescribed as typical beauty standards. Teach yourself what styles, products, tools, and techniques work best for your natural curls as they grow out of your head organically. To really enjoy this daily natural hair journey, accept all the challenges that may come with it and love your tresses, no matter what happens along the way.

Selecting Products for Daily Use

If you already have a routine but need help picking the perfect products, head over to Chapter 7.

Products play a major role in your daily routine. They function to maintain moisture, keep your hair hydrated, maintain your style, or refresh your hair. Maybe you use these products on wash day as well. The practicality of daily products involves helping you maintain your curls between wash days.

It can be a little challenging in the beginning to work out your daily routine. But don't get discouraged.

All you need is time, patience, and some coins to find the perfect cocktail of products. And after you do, your relationship with your hair shifts for the better, and you feel the huge weight of stress lifted off your shoulders. Whether you're a new or experienced natural, you want to find products that work for your hair type and texture. Then, you can figure out a way to fit those products into your lifestyle.

REMEMBER

The more products you use, the more product buildup you get on your hair. So your wash day may come sooner for you versus someone who uses less product.

Not everyone needs to use products every day. Depending on your hair type and texture (flip back to Chapter 3 for help on determining yours), you may need a lot of products or none at all. For example, many people who have Types 2c to 3c hair can freshen up their curls by only misting with water.

Establishing Your Hair Routines

Regardless of whether you set up a morning or night routine, you need to experiment by trying different products at different times to see what works for you. I call the natural hair journey a *journey* for a reason. You need time to embrace your unique curls, break the habit of comparing them to anyone else's, and figure out what works best for you. Trust the process — you can figure it out. Let's begin with the nighttime routine, which you can do before you go to sleep tonight.

Nighttime routine

Establish a nightly routine so that you can reset your hair and maintain volume, curl definition, and length retention until your next wash day. Because wash day comes only once every week or two (flip back to Chapter 4 for a refresher on that idea), your nighttime routine helps keep your hair healthy and looking like you want it to.

Everyone has a slightly different mix of daily products depending your hair texture and type. Through experimentation and trial and error, you can find which ones work for you, and in which combination. But in general, here's a list of lightweight hair moisturizers that you can keep on hand for daily maintenance. You should have at least one or two of these in your beauty supply cabinet for daily use:

>> Oil

>> Cream

>> Mousse

>> Serum

>> Spray

There can be up to four main steps in a nighttime routine, which I talk about in depth in the following section:

1. **Massage**

2. **Moisturize**

3. **Set**

4. **Cover**

WARNING

A bad nightly routine can lead to breakage and a little unruly hair when you wake up in the morning, so take the time for your nightly routine every night.

Massaging your cares away

The first step in your nightly routine — a scalp massage — may sound like a luxury, but it's actually a necessity. Whether your hair is long or short, start off your evening routine with a good 5-minute scalp massage. You can have your boo do it, or you can do it yourself (no oil needed, so it's super easy). It's relaxing and promotes hair growth by stimulating blood circulation. I can't stress enough how beneficial scalp massages are for your hair and scalp, so get to rubbing!

Moisturizing your strands

Lightly apply a moisturizing product to your hair using your fingers. You can rake or comb desired product through your hair. These products can come in oil, spray, cream, or serum form. You don't want anything too heavy because you don't want to soil your scarfs, bonnets, or pillowcases (more on the proper head coverings in the section "Covering your hair," later in this chapter). Choose one that makes your hair feel replenished, nourished, and provides some *slip* (easier it is to move combs or fingers through your hair without friction and tension). Curly hair tends to lose moisture overnight. A lightweight moisturizer can help minimize matting and tangling from friction.

Setting it up

After you moisturize, I suggest putting your hair into a low-manipulation set at night before covering it with a scarf or bonnet. I go into options for protective styling and sets in Chapter 9, but here are a couple of the most common ways you can do this, depending on the length of your hair and how you style it:

» **If you have a twist out:** With a *twist out,* you divide your hair into sections and then twist your wet hair, which helps to keep the curl definition. If you use this style, you may find yourself wanting to retwist a few sections before bedtime that have lost some of their spunk by day three or four.

Locate the section that's beginning to look too frizzy or less defined, and separate it from the rest of your hair. Lightly spray some water directly onto that section (not too much because you want it to dry by the morning). You can apply either the product you used to twist it initially or a different product that you like that helps reset your twists, like oil, gel, or mousse — or even just water. After you retwist those sections, you can leave them as-is or use the pineapple technique that I describe in the following bullet.

If you need more detailed how-to's about twist outs, skip to the section "Styling on the Daily," later in this chapter.

» **If you're rocking a wash-and-go:** You wear your hair in its natural state to show off your curls. When it's time for bed, pull your hair up into a *pineapple,* gently gathering all of your hair to the top of your head and holding it in place by using a loose-fitting hair tie. Leave your curls loose at the top of your head, preventing them from being smashed by your head while you sleep. Pineappling also stretches out your curls, helping to promote volume and curl elongation.

If you want to create more volume and curl elongation, pineapple in four sections. With your fingers, gently separate your hair into four sections, starting by parting your hair down the middle, and then separate each half into two sections so it looks like a cross if someone were to see it from above. Then, pull each section into individual pineapples at the top of your head. This approach stretches out your curls even more (particularly at the crown), and helps you retain your length.

TIP

Depending on your hair type or texture, your curls might not need extra stretching, but you might still want to keep some volume. You can maintain some volume by holding your curls at the top of your head without overstretching them with a hair tie. Just follow these steps to pineapple your hair using a scarf:

1. **Bend over at the waist so that your head is hanging close to the floor and gently smooth your hair towards the top of your head.**

2. **Place your scarf around the back of your head and bring the ends of the scarf to the front of your head.**

3. **Lightly tie the scarf underneath the bangs/fringe area.**

4. **Lift your head up and rearrange the curls in the scarf, if needed.**

TIP

There's no reason why you can't wear your hair in a pineapple wrapped with a decorative scarf for an easy daytime look as shown in Figure 5-2.

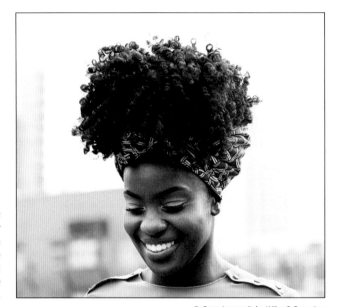

FIGURE 5-2: Pineapple your hair in a decorative scarf for an quick daytime updo.

© Getty Images/John Wiley & Sons, Inc.

Covering your hair

After you moisturize and set your hair, you need to cover your hair. The go-to for naturals include satin or silk scarfs and bonnets (see Figure 5-3). These accessories can best preserve your curls overnight because they reduce friction. As an alternative, a satin or silk pillowcase can keep your hair in great condition while you sleep. For more information on nighttime accessories, see Chapter 6.

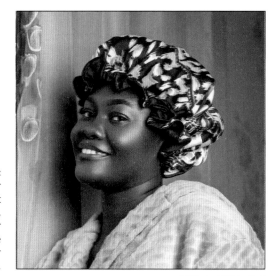

FIGURE 5-3:
A silk or
satin bonnet
(shown),
scarf, or
pillowcase are
must-haves for
naturalistas.

TIP

You can use a scarf and bonnet together — a scarf to hold your hair in place and a bonnet to keep your curls completely covered.

Morning routine

Your morning routine should keep your style looking fresh and get you ready to take on your day. Before you get into that routine, you may need a few things handy:

>> Afro pick

>> Spray bottle filled with lukewarm water

>> Creamy or spray leave-in conditioner

>> Curl-enhancing products

>> Pomade or gel

>> Edge control

>> Small bristle brush

>> Light oil to rub on or an oil mist to finish

REMEMBER

Finding your ideal routine requires experimenting. You may need all these items or just one or two. Play around with the products until you get your desired results. You can hop over to Chapter 7 if you need detailed information about or help choosing specific products.

Once you are ready to style, remove your scarf or bonnet. If you used a pineapple technique, take it down and shake out your hair. You may need to gently pull and separate your hair to get it back into shape. At this point, you can decide whether you need to apply a leave-in or curl-enhancing product to enhance your curls, or if you're happy with your curls as they are.

REMEMBER

Not all hair needs all products and tools. For example, many people who have Types 2c to 3c hair can freshen up their curls by only misting with water. If you have Type 4 hair, you may need to spray your hair with a lot of water first, and then use your products and finger coil to redefine your curls.

After you're happy with your curl pattern, you can use an afro pick at your roots to bring back fullness and volume. Don't comb through your curls with the pick because that creates too much frizz and ruins your curls. Focus on the roots, gently pulling away from the scalp. After you get your shape where you want it and your curls are poppin', grab some edge control, pomade, or gel, and use a brush to help gently tame your hairline.

To finish it all up, grab some oil to spray or smooth onto your hair to seal the cuticles and add some shine. Give yourself a quick wink in the mirror, and you're good to go.

Styling on the Daily

You might be wondering why I would discuss styling in a chapter about routines. I want you to start thinking about how your hairstyles will affect your nighttime and morning routines.

You can style natural hair in countless ways. From twist outs to blowouts, curls come with unmatched versatility. Whether you're a new or experienced natural, enjoy the freedom of exploring your beautiful texture. Play around with different styles (see Figure 5-4).

Back in the day, the afro was one of the only real representations of natural hair. For the most part, everyone looked the same, with a few variations when it came to size. The afro was always full and perfectly symmetrical, having little to no curl definition, created by barbers and stylists by using precision cutting. Although the perfect afro can never go out of style, nowadays, many naturals want more of an organic, loose, and carefree style. They seek curl definition and elongation.

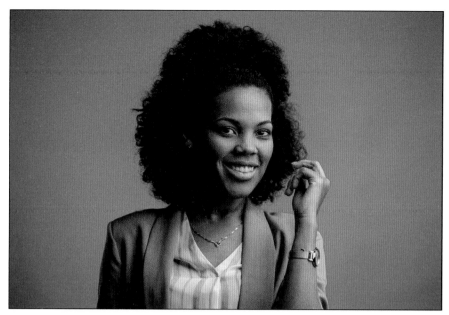

FIGURE 5-4:
Restyle a wash-and-go into a half updo.

Today, everyone wants to look different. We crave individuality. The uniform look is a trend of the past. People lean more towards choosing styles that work with their own personality, face shape, and hair texture and type. Many naturalistas want styles that speak to their unique personal stories and allow them to express themselves without opposition or limits. We should celebrate how far we've come and take full advantage of this new era. Again, play around with different styles — and most of all, have fun.

Although I definitely want you to have fun trying new styles and trends, keep in mind these two main rules when selecting any style:

>> **The foundation of achieving any hairstyle is healthy hair.** Often, you see images of your favorite celebrity or influencer on TV, in magazines, or online rocking a style that you want to try. But remember, as observers, we don't know anything about their haircare regimen. We tend to focus on the style and forget about haircare. That's a recipe for disaster. Always take the time to keep your hair healthy first, and then you can rock any style you desire.

>> **The primary way to maintain healthy hair is by getting a haircut.** Whether it's a designer cut or getting your split ends trimmed, avoiding haircuts can lead to damage and limit your hairstyle options.

TIP

My clients assume that with natural hair, they don't need a cut as often. Quite the contrary. Although natural hair is stronger, it can be just as dry as chemically treated hair. Dry hair tends to have split ends. These split ends can travel up the hair shaft, causing damage. Refreshing your cut or regularly trimming your ends prevents unnecessary damage and enhances your style options.

Be sure to head over to Chapters 9 and 10 for a complete rundown of style ideas and how to create them.

Playing around with twists

Twists are go-to styles for many naturals. Many people incorporate twists into their daily routines, and you can achieve them fairly easily without professional help. When you decide to twist your hair, start your twist set with wet, clean, conditioned hair, and use products that hold and enhance moisture and shine. Then, after you're done twisting, let your hair air dry or sit under a dryer until your hair is completely dry. Here are a few different twist sets and what hair type they work best for (flip back to Chapter 3 if you want a reminder about different hair types):

>> **Comb-twist:** To create a *comb-twist* (also known as *single-twist*), use a small-tooth comb to part the hair into small, symmetrical sections. Grab each section with the end of the comb and twist the hair into small, cylinder-shaped curls. After the hair is completely dry, you can leave it as-is, or you can increase the number of curls by separating the twist two or more times. Comb-twists work best for short hair that falls into Types 3b to 4c.

>> **Flat twist:** To make flat twists, create a flat twist similar to how you create a French braid or cornrow, but use two sections of strands rather than three. Chapter 9 goes into more detail about this technique. Depending on how much definition you want, you can go with six to ten rows. The more rows, the smaller the twist, giving you the most curl definition. Fewer rows give you a looser curl pattern. You can leave your hair in rows of flat twist after they are dry, or you can separate and fluff when dry. You can twist it all the way to the ends, or use a small flexi-rod or perm rod to secure the ends.

>> **Two-strand twist:** With two-strand twists, you take two sections of hair and wrap them around each other in the same direction from the roots all the way to the ends. Two-strand twist works for all hair types, but in particular, it aids in curl definition and elongation for Types 4a to 4c. You can do as many twists as you want, depending on how you want your hair to look. You can leave as-is after they are dry or separate the twists when dry for a twist out.

» **Finger twist:** Do finger twists by simply winding a small section of your hair around your index finger in the direction of its natural curl pattern. After the twists are dry, separate them to multiply your curls and fluff, as desired.

Giving your hair a break from styling

I go more into protective styling in Chapter 9, but I have thoughts that I want to share here because you can make protective styling a part of your daily routine. In my opinion, protective styles have been abused over the years. Naturalistas should use protective styles to protect and preserve their curls for a certain amount of time but many use those same styles as a crutch or bad habit that causes more harm than protection to their hair.

WARNING

Protective styles are supposed to give your hair a break from harsh elements in the environment and manipulation from daily styling, allowing your hair to thrive and grow without interruption. Unfortunately, instead of being patient and taking the time to nourish and really get to know their hair texture, many people use these styles as quick fixes, which can lead to more damage, like breakage and traction alopecia. More about that in Chapter 9.

A few popular protective style options include braids, faux locs/twists, sew-in weaves, and wigs. However, the style you choose shouldn't cause issues with your hair; the way you or your stylist executes the style and how long you keep the style in before you get it redone or taken out can definitely cause issues.

Chapter **6**

Keeping Your Hair Healthy

A re "bad hair days" really a thing? Well, for some people, they are, and they can be very annoying. I know a "bad hair day" is often just a figure of speech, but no one wants to start their day feeling less than confident or insecure because they just can't get their hair to act right. But if you don't handle natural and curly hair with proper care, it becomes prone to damage and bad hair days become the norm.

The fact that you're reading this book clearly shows that you're up for the challenge, so start with concentrating on the health of your hair. Your curls require that you give them focus and time to help them look and feel their best. Too often, people focus on the length of their hair when they should always focus on maintaining healthy hair, regardless of length. With healthy strands, you have no limits when it comes to styling your hair. This chapter gives you the knowledge to help you tweak your hair care routine when needed and maintain your healthy curls effortlessly.

Keeping Your Curls Moisturized

Back in the day, a lot of Black folks rocked a Jheri curl. If you're Gen-Z, you may have no idea what I'm talking about. Just do a quick web search for "Jheri curl" on your smartphone to see a photo. (If your phone is all the way across the room, allow me to give you the basic gist: A Jheri curl is a chemical process that results in a curly, wavy hairstyle that almost always looks glossy or damp.)

Back when everyone wore a Jheri curl, myself included, I noticed how quickly Jheri-curled hair grew and how it retained length so well. Let me tell you why. Those of us with Jheri curls had hair that was always super moisturized — practically wet. Even though we went through a long chemical process to achieve this style, the products that we used for daily maintenance were highly moisturizing and kept hair hydrated the entire day, leaving the hair feeling somewhat wet or greasy to touch. It sometimes got to the point where you could leave a big grease spot on someone's couch if you happen to doze off for a few minutes. (Thank God those days are long gone.)

Each day, we used gels, creams, and sprays filled with an ingredient called glycerin. *Glycerin* (also called glycerol, or the British spelling and pronunciation, glycerine) is a nontoxic, natural humectant that attracts and maintains moisture in your hair and scalp, and can help prevent breakage (more on humectants in Chapter 7). Although no studies have shown that glycerin actually stimulates hair growth, it contributes to scalp health and overall hair health because it's one of the most effective humectants. Hair grows longer faster because the glycerin reduces breakage. Glycerin is still found in a plethora of natural hair products today, but hair product manufacturers have reformulated it to minimize that wet, greasy feeling.

TIP

The benefits of synthetic glycerin have recently decreased in regards to the hair in certain climates. I suggest that you look for organic or natural glycerin instead.

REMEMBER

Why these history lessons? I'll tell you why — because I can't stress enough how important moisture is for maintaining healthy hair. Whether you use a product that has glycerin listed as one of the first three ingredients or you infuse Chebe powder into your favorite natural hair treatment, history has proven over and over again, if you want long, healthy, natural hair, you have to play by the moisture rules.

In Chapter 7, you can find a ton of detail about how and why to hydrate your hair, and you can also get the rundown on the best ingredients and products. But here are a few quick tips for keeping your hair moisturized:

>> **Research the ingredients listed on the labels of your products.** Several products on the market contain harsh chemicals. These products perform well, but over time, they can dry out and damage your hair.

>> **Select products that have water listed as one of the first three ingredients on the label.** To have moisturized hair, it has to be hydrated. And you can't have true hydration if you don't involve water.

THE POWER OF CHEBE POWDER

For centuries, the Basara tribe of Chad, Africa has used a powerful product called Chebe powder that's known to help folks grow natural hair way past their waistlines. Chebe powder is completely natural, made from a mixture of lavender croton, cloves, cherry seeds, and resin tree sap. This powder mixed with water and coconut oil creates a clay-like substance that Chad women apply to their hair once or twice a week, leaving it on for at least one and a half to two hours (even longer when possible). Like glycerin, no studies have shown that Chebe powder stimulates hair growth, but Chadians believe that because of its intensely nourishing, strengthening and — most of all — hydrating and moisture-retaining powers, the Chebe powder leaves their hair feeling stronger, with enhanced growth from length retention. From the pictures I've seen, I definitely think they're on to something.

>> **Figure out your porosity level.** Your porosity level affects how much your hair retains moisture, which means it also affects how you should moisturize your hair (for a refresher on porosity, jump back to Chapter 2).

>> **Use oils or the LOC method to seal in moisture.** LOC stands for leave-in conditioner, oil, and cream. When you seal your hair, you lock moisture into the strand. Flip back to Chapter 4 for a refresher on the LOC method.

>> **Apply conditioner, deep conditioner, or a hair mask every wash day.** Never skip this step. Conditioners feed your hair the nourishment it needs. You can never over-condition your hair. If you want to review wash-day deets, go back to Chapter 4. Just remember to follow a regular cleansing routine because buildup from conditioner can potentially weigh your hair down.

>> **Depending on your hair type or texture, shampoo only once or twice a week.** Shampooing too often can dry out your hair. If you need it, you can find the 411 on hair texture and type back in Chapter 3.

>> **Be mindful of the elements, especially sun exposure.** You may need to switch up your products, depending on the season (for help with picking the right product, skip ahead a smidge to Chapter 7).

>> **Sleep with satin or silk hair coverings or pillowcases.** Satin or silk fabrics help your hair retain moisture, whereas other fabrics pull moisture from your hair.

>> **Minimize heat as much as possible.** Excessive heat dries out your hair and decreases curl definition.

>> **Get to know how your prescribed medications affect your hair by asking your doctor.** Several medications, such as high blood pressure meds, can dry out your hair and your skin.

>> **Stay consistent with your night and morning routine.** Your routines not only help to maintain your style between wash days, but also help to preserve your hair. If you want help getting your routine dialed in, flip back to Chapter 5.

>> **Try your best to maintain a healthy, balanced diet.** You know the saying "You are what you eat." It's true! Foods that contain nutrients such as protein, iron, zinc, biotin, vital fatty acids, and/or vitamins A, B, and C can help to keep your hair strong and shiny.

>> **Consult with a professional, if necessary.** Sometimes you feel like you've done everything possible and still can't figure it out what's going on with your hair. Consulting with a licensed hairstylist can point you in the right direction.

Acknowledging Your Environment: Air Pollution, Humidity, and More

You can control a lot when it comes to the health of your hair: eating a balanced diet, staying consistent with your daily hair routines, exercising, and minimizing stress. Unfortunately, you can't do much about the elements within your environment. You can, however, find ways to maintain healthy hair despite the weather. Read on.

Pollution protection

Air pollution is pretty much everywhere — even indoors — every day. Particulate matter, toxins, and even smoke can all add stress to your hair and scalp.

WARNING

Environments that have high levels of pollution can cause some extra buildup. And even though it doesn't happen often, buildup from air pollution can lead to changes in how your hair looks, making it appear lackluster, dull, or dirty. It can also lead to physical effects on the scalp, causing dandruff, itchiness, and irritation. Also, in some severe cases, pollution can even cause hair loss. I haven't seen a situation like that myself, but I've heard and read about it. Keep it in mind if you decide to dig a little deeper into the medical studies on your own.

Now, you don't need to jump online in search of the least-polluted areas and go pack your bags. Honestly, you can't really escape pollution. Instead, use these three simple tips to combat air pollution like a pro, wherever you are:

>> **Don't skip wash day.** Your wash day gives you an opportunity to detoxify your hair and scalp, and get rid of buildup caused by pollution. Applying conditioner, mask, and hydrating treatments boosts your hair's moisture level, making it less vulnerable to environmental elements (no matter what season you're in. I talk more about this in a later section called "Coping with seasonal change".)

>> **Find ways to soften your water.** A large percent of the United States has hard water. Hard water can create a calcium and magnesium buildup on your hair, very much like the coating you find on faucets and showerheads. This buildup can make it difficult for moisture to penetrate the hair itself.

>> **Use hair serums.** Serums protect the surface and the cuticle layer of your hair and give your curls impeccable shine. Most serums are silicone-based — and some silicones get a bad rap because they can cause buildup on your hair over time. But serums aren't water-soluble, and they prevent humidity (which is water) from penetrating your hair. This waterproofing means serums can really help prevent your hair from swelling up in the humid air during the summer.

Hampering humidity

If you live anywhere but the desert, you know what a beast humidity can be. When it comes to humidity, hair tends to have a mind of its own. But why? Well, *humidity* is the measure of the amount of water vapor in the air. Humidity equals water, and water equals moisture. So think of humidity as basically airborne water. Your hair knows water. You use it to do all kinds of things, such as shampoo and restyle your hair. Hair sucks that water right up. When humidity comes around, your hair wants to automatically absorb it all, which can take a toll on most hairstyles.

You probably already check the weather often to find out the temperature outside. But knowing how humid it is outside tells you more about how you should prep your hair before going out. People who live in dry climates, such as Southern California and Las Vegas, don't have to worry so much about how the weather affects their hair. But anywhere the humidity level goes above 50 percent, NOAA (the National Oceanic and Atmospheric Administration) considers it a humid climate. So how do you maintain your curls and natural hair in such conditions? I'm glad you asked.

Because humidity is water, you might think you can't do much to avoid the physical effects it has on your hair. Well, I can offer some tips to help you deal with those steamy, hot summer months.

TIP

Anti-humectant and anti-frizz products can help slow down humidity absorption so that you can maintain your style a little longer in these climates. Products with hold, such as hairspray, gels, and mousses, can help combat humidity by providing a protective layer. Although they can leave your hair feeling a little crunchy, they help reduce the physical effects that humidity can have on your hair. And throughout the day, the humidity can help release that crunchy cast.

And I need to offer a little loving reality check for you. If you're outdoors for a long period of time in an all-time-high humidity level (see Figure 6-1), you have a very high chance of your hair becoming a little fussy. If that's the case, embrace it. Don't let a little frizz ruin your moment. Have fun with it and continue to *get your entire life*. I promise you that no one worth having in your life is going to judge you because your hair is reacting naturally to the elements. Personally, I love to see curls tossed in a dash of humidity. The messiness looks effortless, sexy, and fashionable, in my opinion.

But if you want to fight the good fight against your hair reacting to humidity, you can always do one of the following:

>> **Cover it up.** Wear scarfs or satin-lined hats or caps to keep your hair covered while you're outdoors.

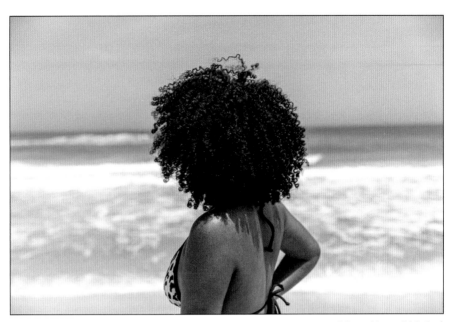

FIGURE 6-1:
Don't fight
humidity,
embrace it!

>> **Use protective styles.** Wear crochet styles, Bantu knots, or different types of braids during the summer months.

>> **Stay away from heat styling.** The amount of heat you need to try to keep your hair straight can definitely cause heat damage. Instead, pull your hair into an updo or a chic, low-bun ponytail.

>> **Rock an afro.** You don't have to worry about frizz with a 'fro.

>> **Keep your hair struggles to yourself.** Just lock yourself up in the house and cover all the mirrors until the weather forecast shows the humidity levels lower than 50 percent. I'm kidding, don't do that. But — and I say this with love — no one wants to hear you complaining about humidity and your hair while everyone's out having some fun under the sun. Take the right precautions or just keep it to yourself, sweetie.

Coping with seasonal change

Can seasonal changes affect the health of your hair? It absolutely can! You can read about the impact that pollution and humidity can have on your hair and scalp in the preceding sections, but drastic temperature changes can also have some challenging effects. Just like you switch up the way you dress when seasons change, you also may need to switch up your hair routine.

To be honest with you, all curls aren't created equal — which means you might not even need to change your hair routine when seasons change. I just want to give you as much information as possible in case you notice a difference in your hair when the weather changes drastically.

Summer

When summer arrives, the main environmental change to pay close attention to besides humidity (discussed in the preceding section) involves the increasingly powerful UV rays. Depending on their intensity, UV rays can wreak havoc on your curls. When you start to expose your hair to more sun and the UV rays are at their strongest, your hair can become dry, brittle, and rough to touch. UV rays might also reduce the protein in your hair because they lift the cuticle, which causes holes to form in the hair shaft. Then, you lose keratin, making your hair more prone to breakage. Much like bleach, UV rays can oxidize your hair pigment over time, causing your color to fade.

Though you can't feel it, your hair can sunburn, just like your skin. It has the same impact as excessive exposure to high heat tools. It gets dry and damaged. Did you know that some hair products contain sunscreen? Yep, it's a real thing and worth adding to your summer routine. The sun's rays can not only do a number on your hair, but also irritate your scalp. Hair products labeled as having SPF include UV-filtering ingredients that protect the hair and the scalp. With any protective product you choose, be sure to check the manufacturer's instructions for proper usage.

Throughout the summer months, stock up on products that can help you protect your hair against extreme heat and harsh UV rays:

>> **Heat protectants:** Act as a barrier between your hair and the heat/UV source, which helps reduce heat damage effectively. They often come in the form of a serum, spray, or cream that you leave in your hair when it's either damp or dry.

>> **Certain leave-in conditioners:** Some of these products also provide heat protection. You can use these in addition to your serums, sprays, and creams to add an extra layer of protection.

>> **Shea butter and oils:** If you seek a more natural approach for heat protection, shea butter and oils (such as almond oil, coconut oil, and avocado oil) can help protect your hair from heat damage. Just apply a little all over your hair before going outside.

And for swimmers and beach bunnies, chlorine and salt water can dry out your hair as much as the sun can. Wear a swim cap to protect your curls while you're swimming. Some naturalistas also like to put conditioner on their hair before swimming in chlorine to protect their curls.

Winter

During the winter, heavy wind and bitter cold air can pull moisture out of your hair, so you definitely want to stay on top of your hydration and protein treatments to keep your hair moisturized and strong.

But even more than strong hair, you probably need to focus on your scalp during this season. For many years, I've witnessed more itchy and flaky scalps in the wintertime than any other season. You create the perfect storm when you go between the harsh cold air outside and the dry heat inside, putting extra stress on your hair and increasing dryness on your scalp. Your hair responds with static and frizz, and your scalp becomes itchy and flaky. These flakes could just be from a dry scalp or from a more accelerated issue such as dandruff.

If you start to notice itchiness and flaking during the winter months, you should definitely apply hot oil treatments more often and use anti-dandruff shampoos that nourish the scalp and clear up flakes. During the winter, you also want to amp up your moisture by using steam treatments, in addition to your conditioners and mask. (For more about steam treatments, visit Chapter 4.)

Also, make sure your hair is completely dry before you go outside. Although I encourage air drying during the summer, going out with wet or damp hair in the winter can stress your curls and just feel extremely uncomfortable. Additionally, avoid unlined knitted and wool hats, scarves, and coat collars. The friction from rough material can snap and break your curls. I can't even begin to tell you how many times my clients have experienced excessive snagging with wool materials.

TIP

Line your hats, scarves, and coat collars with a thin silk or satin scarf to protect your hair from friction. Or buy them readymade.

Preserving Your Beautiful Curls

Maintaining healthy hair essentially preserves your curls — and it's no secret that you need effort, knowledge, time, and patience to properly care for natural curly hair. Getting to know your hair, using quality ingredients, finding the safest tools for styling, or sticking to your daily routine and wash day can all help you get a healthy head of curls. You may find getting the hang of curl care challenging in the beginning, but practice makes perfect. Give yourself time to figure it out; before you know it, you'll be preserving your beautiful curls easily.

Trimming your hair

The shrinkage is real — and if you're like many naturals, you have hair growth and length retention as continual goals throughout your hair journey, so the last thing a lot of people want to do is trim their hair. If you want to grow your hair into a longer style, watch out because you can easily become slightly obsessed and a little too attached to that goal. If you focus on always adding length, you might overlook and neglect your fragile split ends because you mistake them for actual length. But in fact, split ends don't give you any actual length. If you're avoiding regular trims because you don't want to let go of perceived length, you risk damaging the healthy part of your strands.

Split ends happen when the ends of your strands become fragile, brittle, and dry. They start to fray and split, and they eventually break off. When you neglect to trim your ends, the frayed, split ends can travel up the hair shaft, causing more damage and breakage. You have to get rid of that dead weight and allow your hair to grow evenly. Excessive heat, poor hair care habits, daily manipulation from your hair care and styling techniques, exposure to harsh weather conditions, lack of moisture, hair coloring, and naturally aged strands can all cause split ends.

Here are a few signs to keep an eye out for so that you can recognize when you have split ends that need trimming:

>> The ends of your hair look lackluster and dull, and they feel crunchy and hard.

>> Your hair gets more tangled than it usually does and takes longer to detangle.

>> You start to notice knots at the bottom of your strands.

>> Your curls just don't look quite the same, and you have trouble getting your hair to hold a style.

>> Your hair breaks off easily, making it look like your hair isn't growing.

Now, I know you're probably expecting some type of DIY advice on trimming your own hair at home. Sorry, not sorry: If you want that advice, head over to YouTube university. As a professional hairstylist, I really can't recommend ways to trim your hair on your own. I just haven't seen many success stories. I don't even trim my own hair because I personally believe that proper hair trimming should be left in the hands of an outside professional.

Schedule a trim at least every three months if you're natural from root to ends. That's approximately four times a year. If you stay on schedule and adapt to good healthy hair habits, you'll notice your stylist removing less hair each time.

TIP

If you're growing out your relaxer, schedule a trim every six to eight weeks. The relaxed ends are more fragile and can split more frequently.

Employing low-manipulation techniques

Hair is very delicate, and how you handle it daily affects how it grows and retains length. *Low manipulation* involves handling your curls with gentle and patient hands. By employing low-manipulation techniques, you can maintain healthy hair because you put minimal stress on your strands. These techniques create styles that require less pulling, combing, and touching, in general. Manipulate your hair less by creating a low-manipulation style. After you get that style done, you can leave your hair alone, practically going hands-free for a few days — even as long as a week — depending on the style.

TIP

Especially if you have very fine hair or your hair tends to be fragile, practicing low-manipulation techniques can help you maintain the health of your hair.

First, to set yourself up for low manipulation, moisturize your hair well and seal it with a light oil to enhance *slippage* (the more slip a product gives your hair, the easier it is to move combs or fingers through your hair without friction and tension). This preparation creates a great foundation for low-manipulation styles. After you style it, you just need some edge control or gel to touch up your hairline throughout the week (jump to Chapter 7 if you need help picking products).

You have several low-manipulation styles to choose from that you can wear at least one week out of the month, when you want to keep your hands out of your hair for a bit (see Part 4 for more on how to do these styles):

>> Ponytails

>> High or low buns

>> Updos

>> Bantu knots

>> Cornrows and braids

>> Crochet styles

When thinking of low-manipulation hair care, consider adding a few steps to your routine. These steps might take a little more time, but the benefits are worth it in the end:

>> **On wash day, if your hair isn't too tangled, divide your hair into small sections.** Use your fingers to gently detangle, rather than brushes or combs.

When using brushes and combs to detangle, people often rush and forget to be gentle. Using your fingers encourages you to slow down and approach detangling more gently because you can actually feel your strands.

>> **When it's time to shampoo, section your hair and shampoo each section individually.** Depending on the length and density of your hair, you may want to divide it into four or six sections. Dividing your hair up makes it easier to manage and minimizes the chances of your hair tangling back up after shampooing, so you don't need to detangle again.

>> **While applying conditioners or masks, work in sections and thoroughly saturate your hair.** Let your hair sit under indirect heat from a hooded dryer or steamer for a few minutes before combing the conditioner through. The heat helps soften your hair, making it easier to comb through any additional tangles.

TIP

During your low-manipulation week, air dry your hair to reduce the pulling and tugging you do while using a hair dryer.

Using heat (or not)

"To heat or not to heat?" That is the question. But it's not just any question. It's probably one of the most-asked questions by curl-friends during their natural hair journey — and understandably so. Heat damage is permanent; you can't do a thing to reverse it. You just have to wait until your new hair grows in to replace the damaged hair. Excessive heat can strip moisture out of your strands and permanently straighten your hair like relaxers do — except relaxers use chemicals to do it immediately, versus doing it slowly without chemicals over time. The great thing about using heat versus chemicals is that the heat lets you retain more volume and fullness. The downside is that using heat to straighten is not as deep and permanent, so if you go into a humid climate, for example, you may see some curl come back.

WARNING

Although you can treat heat damage and reduce hair loss, most of the time, the structural change to your curl pattern that happens is here to stay when that happens. Other times, you can get back some of your curls with proper bonding treatments. Eventually, your new hair will come out undamaged.

But simply using heat on healthy hair doesn't automatically mean that the heat you use leaves your hair damaged. Of course, you might experience heat damage if you use too high heat for too long, but you can also totally prevent it. Even if you've had heat damage in the past, it doesn't mean you're going to let it happen to the new hair you're growing.

All heat is not created equal. The hot air from a hood dryer or blow dryer, and the direct heat from a flat iron, wand, or curling iron, exposes your hair to two different types of heat.

Hot air from hood dryers and blow dryers dries the hair by eliminating water gradually over time. You can use dryers to set your hair and for blowouts:

>> **Setting your hair:** When you use dryers to set your hair (via rollers, rods, or diffusers), you typically apply little to no tension on your strands, and the hot air doesn't affect the integrity and structure of your curls.

When using a dryer to set your hair, switch the dryer setting between cool and hot/warm to lock in your set.

>> **Blowouts:** When you use dryers for blowouts, you apply more tension (because you use blow dry brushes, comb attachments, and stretching). A little tension doesn't do damage to your hair, but because wet hair is fragile, too much tension mixed with heat can weaken the shaft and loosen your curl pattern.

For tips on blowing out your hair like a pro, head over to Chapter 9.

With flat irons, wands, and curling irons, the electrical current travels through the cord to the device, heating the element (the iron or wand). When you place your hair on the surface of these tools, you expose it to a direct heat source, which is much hotter than the air from a dryer. But if you have the right knowledge, tools, and techniques, you can successfully use these direct heat tools without causing damage.

If you do a quick search on the Internet for "proper heat for my hair texture," all kinds of articles and quotes pop up, stating that your hair can withstand a temperature of 450 degrees Fahrenheit (232 degrees Celsius) before burning. But because everyone doesn't have the same head of hair, you have to select a temperature that's right for your particular hair type and texture.

I can suggest ranges, such as

>> **Fine hair:** 275 to 300 degrees Fahrenheit (121–149 degrees Celsius)

>> **Normal hair:** 350 to 375 degrees Fahrenheit (177–191 degrees Celsius)

>> **Coarse hair:** 385 to 410 degrees Fahrenheit (204–232 degrees Celsius)

But to figure out the right temperature for your hair, just start off with moderate heat and work your way up until you achieve your desired finish. Temperatures above 430 degrees Fahrenheit (221 degrees Celsius) are typically way too much heat for most hair textures if you want to preserve your curls.

If you want to preserve your curls, heat style it, at most, two to six times a year, depending on your hair texture. Save it for those special occasions or events. If you have super fine, fragile hair, you probably want to ditch direct heat completely.

For tips on what to look for in a blow dryer and a flat iron, flip to Chapter 8.

Caring for your color-treated hair

Even though I don't recommend coloring or bleaching your own hair, you can do several things at home to help maintain healthy hair after you receive professional coloring services (see Figure 6-2):

>> **On wash day, use shampoos designed for color-treated hair.** Normal shampoos, particularly ones that contain sulfate, can diminish the vibrancy of your new color.

>> **Deep condition on every wash day and sit under a steamer while you have the conditioner on your hair.** If you read Chapter 4, you know I love steam treatments, especially for color-treated hair, because it enhances the longevity of your color. Plus, steam treatments really improve the overall health of your hair.

>> **Use leave-in conditioners regularly.** You really can't over-condition your hair. Color-treated hair is typically thirsty because the process of coloring removes pigment, which causes moisture loss. Plus, the chemicals cause dehydration. Your hair will thank you for all the extra hydration.

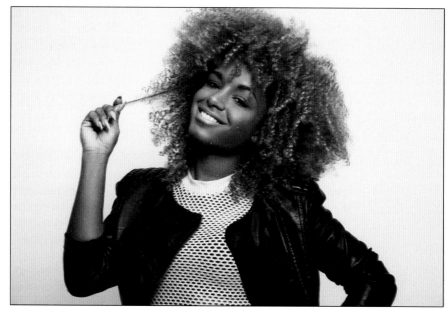

FIGURE 6-2:
With the right shampoo, conditioners, and routines, you can maintain your color-treated hair at home.

© Anastasia/Adobe Stock

>> **Always style by using the LOC method.** LOC stands for leave-in, oil, conditioner. For a refresher on that technique, flip back to Chapter 4. If you moisturize your hair when you style it, you can keep your colored hair soft, shiny, and less prone to breakage.

>> **Use heat protectant regularly.** Sun rays and direct heat from styling tools can strip permanent color out of your hair. Using a heat protectant adds a protective barrier between your hair color and the heat.

>> **Try to implement low-manipulation hairstyles for at least one to two weeks out of the month.** Natural hair is naturally fragile — and color-treated natural hair can be even more fragile because it's going through a chemical process that weakens it. Low-manipulation hairstyles can help keep those fragile strands intact.

Selecting your nighttime accessories

Two of the best fabrics to use when you want to protect and preserve your natural and curly hair are silk and satin. Using silk or satin bonnets, scarves, durags, and pillowcases over your hair while you're sleeping keeps those curls, braids, and waves intact. Unlike cotton that combats our hair with its raised texture, fabrics such as silk and satin complement our hair textures because they are smooth, so they create practically no friction and therefore don't aggravate your curls. Without friction, your curls can maintain their shape and moisture levels. As an added bonus, silk and satin are cooling fabrics that help prevent sweating overnight.

WARNING

Aside from the rough texture, cotton also strips moisture out of your hair and can leave your curls all over the place and feeling dry and brittle in the morning.

Now that you know these miraculous fabrics, the following sections discuss the pros and cons of various hair maintenance accessories made of those fabrics.

Bonnets

Bonnets are possibly the most popular unpopular choice for hair protection that you can use. Popular because they are the most effective, least expensive way to protect your curls without compression. And unpopular because the debate about bonnets being worn in public is one that has played out online and on social media for some time now.

The conversation doesn't focus on the practicality of bonnets; instead, it criticizes people for wearing bonnets in public. Some think that wearing bonnets in public represents a lack of self-respect and a loss of pride in how you present yourself. Others think it's nobody's business what anyone else wears on their head.

You can find people on both sides of the fence on this topic, but here's my opinion: I don't have one! Just because someone who looks like you decides to present themselves in a certain way in public doesn't mean they represent you — or a group of people who look like you, for that matter. Do what works for you. Furthermore — and I say this with love — if anyone has the time and energy to focus on how you look in public, when it literally doesn't affect them, they probably need a new hobby. *Bloop!*

Okay, now that I got that off my chest, another tip about bonnets: They have the tendency to slip off while you toss and turn, so purchase one that fits nice and snug (then you don't have to worry about losing it overnight).

Scarves and durags

Scarves and durags both offer great protection and can give your hair some compression, helping keep your curls or waves intact overnight. Most people use hair scarves to help lay their edges down. After you shape your hairline the way you want it, tie a silk or statin scarf over your edges while they dry in place. You can also use a scarf when you're sporting a silky blowout and want to use the wrapping technique at night to keep your hair straight.

Durags are very popular for men, but anyone with shorter hair can use them. They give you the perfect balance of protection and compression when you have waves or braids.

WARNING

The main issue I've noticed when people use scarves and durags is that they often tie them too tightly. When you tie a durag too tightly, you can end up experiencing lightheadedness and headaches. Make sure they feel completely comfortable before you tuck in.

Satin and silk pillowcases

If you don't feel comfortable covering your head at night when you're with your boo, or you just simply want to feel completely free while you recharge, get yourself some satin or silk pillowcases. They feel so pleasant to sleep on, and they give your curls solid protection without making you feel confined. However, if you have a style that needs any compression, pillowcases can't help you. Also, satin and silk pillowcases can cost you, but they're absolutely worth the investment.

Consulting with a Professional

I haven't met many hairstylists who aren't passionate about their craft. We not only love styling and contributing to the illustration of your personal stories, we also find great joy in helping you maintain healthy hair during your hair journey.

With just one glance, we know your hair type and texture, and our creative juices start to flow as we start thinking of ways to style it.

No matter what your situation is, a professional hairstylist is trained to deliver exactly what you want and need — or, at the very least, point you in the right direction to get what you need somewhere else. Whether you're a new natural or transitioning from a relaxer, or you've been working your curls for years, you always want a trusted, experienced hairstylist in your arsenal.

Reasons to bring in a pro

Throughout this book, I emphasize when to consult with a professional hairstylist. Although I offer a plethora of ways to take care of your hair at home, there also comes a time when you need to schedule an appointment with a professional (see Figure 6-3). Here are some reasons to bring in a pro:

» **When it's time for a haircut:** In the section "Trimming your hair," earlier in this chapter, I suggest leaving proper trimming in the hands of a professional. Well, I feel the same way about haircuts. Cutting hair is an artform that requires a lot of knowledge and practice, even with trims. It doesn't matter how easy your favorite influencer makes it look when they "show you how to cut your own hair." Cutting your own hair can be a complete disaster.

» **When you decide to transition from relaxer to natural:** Transitioning hair is very delicate. A pro can create styles and treat your hair so that you can make a more seamless transition.

» **When you want to change your hair color or had an unsuccessful attempt with coloring your hair at home:** Whether you used at-home store-bought color or got your hands on some professional color, you might not end up with the color you expected. Here's a rule of thumb: Whenever you need a chemical service, leave it up to the experts.

» **When you can't figure out the best selection of products to keep your hair moisturized and healthy:** Because so many different people sit in a hairstylist's chair, we get the opportunity to work with all hair types and textures. Professional hairstylists can suggest the best hair products for your unique head of hair.

» **When you can't fix scalp issues with home remedies:** A professional hairstylist can definitely help solve scalp issues, but you might need to book an appointment with a dermatologist for severe cases.

» **When you simply just want to be pampered:** Hairstylists and salons offer a variety of services. Sometimes, you just want to relax and let someone else do all the work.

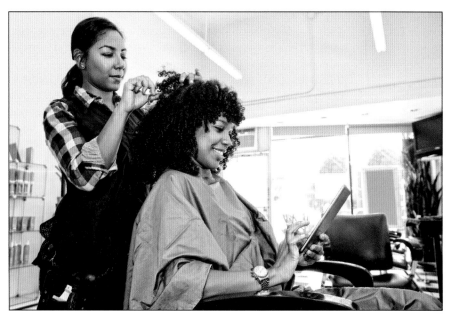

FIGURE 6-3: A licensed hairstylist can provide guidance to properly care for your hair.

Finding the right professional for you

You can easily find a professional hairstylist these days. Literally walk down any commercial business avenue to find a salon on every other block. The challenge comes in finding the right professional for *you*.

Fortunately, over the past 10 to 12 years, natural and curly hair has become the main attraction. More and more people feel encouraged to go natural and show off their curly tresses. Hairstylists all over the globe are taking continuing education courses in hopes of expanding their knowledge about textured hair.

Finding the stylist for you might be as easy as asking your friends. But if you don't have a good curl-friend who has a healthy head of curls and can recommend the hairstylist they go to, how do you find a good natural hairstylist?

I always suggest doing Internet research. Search through Google, Yelp, and different hairstylists' social media accounts. Thankfully, social media platforms such as Instagram and TikTok provide a great way to see exactly what a stylist offers and the types of textures they work with. At whatever social media site you frequent, just type "natural hair" into the search bar and click Search, and a whole host of accounts pop up. If you find an account that features a stylist who talks directly to the camera and posts good weekly tips on natural hair care, you've probably found a legit hairstylist to follow and possibly book an appointment with.

When you find stylists whose online presence you like, create a list. In your list, include stylists who seem to have a wealth of knowledge about natural hair care, post pictures of clients who have curls that look similar to yours, and have a passion for textured hair. After you come up with a solid list (about seven to ten salons), head over to YouTube and search for personal reviews. Just search for the salon or stylist's name plus "reviews," and you might find real reviews from people's experience at that salon or with that stylist.

Search out salons and stylists who specialize in natural and curly hair. In smaller markets, it might be a little harder than it is in big cities, but keep at it. And don't be afraid to ask other naturalistas or people whose hair you admire.

After you gather all the information that you need, check availability. You can simply call the salon where the stylist works or visit the salon's or stylist's website. If their book is wide open, you probably want to think twice and try the next salon on your list. Although you may find it annoying, if they're booked for weeks to months out, that gives you a good indication that the salon has residual clientele, which means people like their work. Grab the first available appointment.

You can schedule your first appointment just as a consultation, where you can ask all the questions I list in the following section. Or if you feel confident in this stylist, you can book a consultation followed by a treatment service. Booking a treatment (like a hot oil or steam or protein treatment) as your first service allows you to have a solid experience with the hairstylist and gives you the opportunity to observe the salon from within before you schedule a cut or style. If you like the experience, congratulations! You found your match. Go shop for a ring and add more services to your next appointment.

You might have different stylist for different services, and there's absolutely nothing wrong with that. Maybe one stylist specializes in treatments and cutting, and another stylist specializes in treatments and coloring. This kind of specialization is totally common in the hair industry, and you can have a back-up stylist you know and trust with your curls.

Good questions to ask during a consultation

Textured hair can be way too fragile to just book an appointment at the most convenient salon that pops up on your web search. When you're looking for a stylist, book a consultation. It can serve almost like a job interview where you can get to know them and their work better. Although many stylists claim to be natural hair experts in an attempt to grow their clientele, a true expert needs to have solid training and experience that you need to know more about. Unfortunately, you can find a lot of misinformed hairstylists out there.

You can have a lot of reasons to look for a new stylist. Maybe you don't have a regular one. Maybe you've outgrown your current one. Maybe your stylist retired. Maybe you're visiting or you've moved to a completely new city or state. Whatever the reason, the hair consultation helps you begin to lay the foundation to build a relationship between you and the stylist.

Naturally (no pun intended), provide pictures of what you want to achieve with your hair, and then hopefully it flows into a transparent conversation that revolves around your hair history, lifestyle and habits, technical aspects of your hair structure, and your hair goals. Cover all of these topics during an initial consultation, and allow the stylist to examine your hair and scalp so that they know exactly what they're getting into with having you as a client. Also, have some questions prepared so that you know exactly what you're getting into with having them as your stylist. How the stylist answers your questions also gives you an opportunity to check the vibes of the salon and stylist.

Here's a list of questions that can help you get to know a hairstylist:

>> Are you a licensed hairstylist?

>> What are your prices, and do they vary based on density, texture, or length?

>> What percentage of your clientele has natural and curly hair?

>> What type of natural and curly hair products do you use?

>> What cutting techniques do you use for curly hair and why?

>> Where can I find pictures of natural hairstyles and haircuts that you've created?

>> What's the state of my overall hair health currently, and can I achieve my goals based on the pictures I've shown you?

>> How long do you estimate it will take for me to achieve what I want, and what can I expect during my natural hair journey?

>> What protective styles are best for my hair journey?

Be clear and upfront about your hair goals and ask assertive questions to get to know the stylist better and what they can offer. Always say what you mean and mean what you say (just don't say it mean!). Your gut's all you got. So, if the energy isn't wright (pun intended!), you don't seem to have a connection, or you just don't feel comfortable, politely leave. Nobody has time for that. That advice goes for both you and the stylist. If you don't have a good fit, just carry on and continue your search until you find the perfect curl pro for you.

REMEMBER

A proper consultation with a new client takes about 30 minutes. Some hairstylists have a consultation fee that compensates them for their time, which they might combine with your first service.

3

The Best Products and Tools for Natural and Curly Hair

Find the right products to keep your hair healthy and looking better than ever.

Use the right tools to maintain your hair and achieve the style you want.

Discover which ingredients to look for or stay away from when selecting hair care products.

IN THIS CHAPTER

» Diving into the importance of water

» Identifying the key types of product ingredients

» Discovering which ingredients should be avoided

» Personalizing product use to your hair type

» Using items you have at home to treat your hair

Chapter **7**

Picking the Perfect Products

Whether you purchase your hair products at your local drugstore, a high-end supplier, or an online retailer — or you make your own with organic ingredients from your kitchen or local grocery — this chapter points you in the right direction while you embark on the search for the best products.

You can find an infinite number of products in the world. So rather than provide you with a catalog or product guide in this chapter, I mainly focus on giving you the ins and outs of the most important ingredients for healthy curls, kinks, and coils. With this information, you can make your own educated choices, wherever and whenever you shop. The ingredients I go over here apply to all hair care and styling products: shampoos, conditioners, hair masks, oils, creams, gels — everything.

I start by highlighting the most important ingredient of all, then I discuss how different ingredients fit into different categories according to their function and features. Next, I detail how to select products with ingredients that work best for your hair texture and which ones you should avoid. I even give you a few DIY tips for turning products you have in your kitchen into hair care wonder treatments.

Plus, I've positively packed this chapter with pro tips that aim to get your natural tresses healthy, hydrated, and styled to the *Gawds!*

Focusing on the Holy Grail of Hair Care

Before I jump into the nitty gritty of which products are best for your particular hair type and texture, let me just say that one ingredient is vital for everyone's hair. It's more important than any other ingredient, no matter what kind of product you use or hair you have on your head. And this holy grail of products for natural and textured hair is also the most accessible: It's water!

REMEMBER

Water is vital to your entire body, and your hair is no exception! If you take only one thing away from this book, make it this: Hydration is the key to healthy hair, and nothing is more hydrating than water. The ultimate goal is to keep as much water in your hair as possible.

It's important to note that natural and curly hair can be extra prone to dryness and frizz. It's harder for *natural scalp oils* (or sebum) to travel from the roots to the ends to entirely coat curly hair strands, which is not the case for straight or slightly wavy hair. Sebum must travel around the twists and bends in curly hair and often coats only a small portion of the hair shaft. That portion is typically closer to the scalp. This is why conditioning and products play a big role in keeping your hair hydrated and moisturized.

Mastering your hair's water level: Hydrating and moisturizing

There are two parts to successfully mastering your hair's water level. Although they might appear to be the same thing to the untrained eye, they do have their differences:

» **Hydrating your hair:** Exposing your hair to enough water so that it penetrates the inside of the hair fiber. The porosity of your hair can affect how much water penetrates your hair, so everyone has different hydration needs. For a refresher on hair porosity, jump back to Chapter 2.

» **Moisturizing your hair:** Locking water into your hair shaft by softening the hair shaft and sealing in nutrients.

Hydrating your hair is pretty straightforward: Drench your hair with water, making sure the hair is completely saturated. I suggest running the water through your hair for at least 3 to 4 minutes, either in the shower or bath, or in any other way you can expose your head to a lot of water. The longer you soak your hair, the more water your hair follicles absorb. Hydrating your hair doesn't get much easier than that, right? Well, because you can't live in water — and weeklong showers are generally frowned upon by polite society — eventually the water evaporates and your hair dries up. You just can't surround your hair with water 24/7. So you need moisturizing.

In a nutshell, moisturizing is applying products on the outside of your hair to help it retain as much water as possible. You can find all sorts of products for moisturizing — and some for hydrating, as well.

Before I give you the product rundown (see the section "Exploring the Basics of Vital Hair Care Ingredients," later in this chapter), I want to make sure you know how to get a read on your hair's hydration status (which I talk about in the following section). You can most easily remember the difference between hydrating and moisturizing by the fact that hydrating happens on the inside of the hair, but moisturizing happens on the outside.

Checking in on your hair's hydration situation

Before you go loading up your shopping cart with all kinds of products, take a second to figure out just how thirsty your locs currently are. Checking your hair's hydration level is, in many ways, intuitive. Look for these signs of possible dehydration:

>> Your hair looks dull and lacks shine.

>> Your hair feels coarse and not soft to the touch.

>> Your hair breaks easily and does not hold up to pressure.

>> Your curls look frizzy and messy, and not plump and defined.

The preceding list doesn't include every sign of hair dehydration; it just gives you a few quick clues to look for.

REMEMBER

Aside from plain old water, water-based products are your hair's best friend. Nothing is more vital to healthy hair than keeping the right level of water in it. When you select your shampoo, conditioner, and any type of treatment products, always look at the labels and choose products that list water (or aqua) as one of the first three ingredients.

Styling products that contain water can also add to your hair health, but unlike treatment products, water doesn't have to appear in the top three ingredients of styling products.

Exploring the Basics of Vital Hair Care Ingredients

If you're reading this section, you've probably determined that your hair is in need of some hydration love. But with thousands of products on the shelves in stores and online, how do you know which products to choose? How do you even start? Say no more — I'm here to help you choose the right products, and you may soon be wondering how you ever lived without them.

REMEMBER

Use the amount and type of product that makes the most sense for your hair type.

On the labels of your shampoo, conditioner, hair mask, or any other hair care product, you can find the ingredients list. I know that sometimes the ingredients list can be so long that you feel overwhelmed and confused. But really, you only need to know how to identify the most key ingredients and their functions. These ingredients fall into three basic categories:

>> **Humectants:** Hydrators that attract water from the air and transfer it into your hair

>> **Emollients:** Moisturizers; the oils (think shea butter, argan, and jojoba) that soften, smooth, and detangle your hair

>> **Occlusives:** Also moisturizers; typically thick, and you can use them to seal in water

You can probably understand and identify humectants easily enough. These substances penetrate your hair and add moisture to it. You might find emollients and occlusives a little confusing because they have similar properties and uses, and many ingredients can work as both emollients and occlusives. Both emollients and occlusives moisturize the hair on the outside, but unlike emollients, occlusives also lock in your hair's internal moisture by applying a seal to the hair shaft.

Sometimes, products contain ingredients from all three categories. Leave-in-conditioners, for example, very commonly have ingredients from each category. Although each category of ingredients has its own unique properties, you may want to use a product that has all three if you have dry or damaged hair because you can hydrate, moisturize, and seal your hair all at once.

If you do choose to use singular products, the order of application is

1. **Humectants**
2. **Emollients**
3. **Occlusives**

Remember, whether you use these products daily, weekly, or monthly depends on your personal hair care needs (turn back to Chapter 4 if you need a refresher on hair care basics).

TIP

When you're shopping for products and reading labels, consider how many products you want to use in the end. Are you a person who loves as many products as possible, or do you prefer to keep things simple? Select your hair care accordingly! And be honest with yourself because if you end up dreading your hair care routine because it's either too boring or too *extra*, you won't do it.

Humectants

Humectants are the foundation of hydrating products. If your hair is dry or damaged because of dehydration, get some humectants into your hair, stat. They bring water into your hair from the air to help

>> Soften your hair and retain its curl.

>> Add elasticity and bounce to your hair.

>> Fortify your hair against the heat, wind, and other elements.

A ton of ingredients fall into this category, so if you're super interested, definitely spend some time on the web reading more about humectants. You'll probably find some ingredients you've heard of before, but you might find some you haven't. A few common ingredients that fall under this category include

>> Glycerin

>> Hyaluronic acid

>> Proteins (such as collagen or keratin)

>> Sugars (such as glucose and fructose)

>> Panthenol

Because humectants take water out of the air to hydrate your hair, their performance is very dependent on the environment. They are most effective in *neutral environments* — climates that are neither extremely humid nor extremely dry.

WARNING

In climates that are humid, humectants may bring in too much water, essentially overhydrating your hair. Your hair shafts become bloated, and then your hair gets sticky, big, and frizzy — the exact opposite of what you want to achieve. On the other hand, in climates that are dry, humectants can make your hair even drier because they can't pull any water from the air. When that happens, humectants pull water up from deep within the hair shaft, which just makes things even worse.

So what do you do if you live in a very dry or very humid place? Make sure your hair care product also includes moisturizers such as occlusives or emollients (which I talk about in the following sections).

Emollients

After your hair has enough water inside it thanks to humectants, emollients, and occlusives are the ingredients that act as moisturizers to lock in that hydration.

I want to first dispel the myth that emollients hydrate your hair — they don't. Rather, emollients help your hair retain the water that it already contains. You can use these oils and butters to smooth, fill in, and coat the outside of your hair with a film. This film coats the hair so that the occlusives can seal in the water. Emollients also bring back the oil to the hair before you seal your hair with occlusives.

>> Help soften your hair strands.

>> Keep your hair from tangling.

>> Increase *slippage,* which is exactly what it sounds like: the ability of your hair strands to slip easily around each other. When you have good slippage, you can more easily maintain your curl pattern and prevent frizz.

Here are a few common emollients that you can look for in your product ingredients lists (you can find more information about them in the section "Oils," later in this chapter):

>> Shea butter

>> Jojoba oil

>> Dimethicone (silicone oil)

>> Cetrimonium chloride

For additional info on emollients, check out the sidebar "Fatty alcohols," in this chapter.

Not only do emollients show up as ingredients in shampoos and conditioners, you can also use them as standalone products. Try them after you shampoo and condition, right before you style — or to refresh your style between wash days. For more on using them, flip back to Chapter 4.

Occlusives (a.k.a. sealants)

Occlusives (also known as *sealants*) are similar to emollients. Occlusive butters and oils have a thick consistency that

» Serves primarily to lock or seal in moisture.

» Prevents water from escaping from your hair.

» Can be too greasy, but not if you use lighter options.

You can often find occlusives paired with humectants in hair care products to counteract dryness caused by the glycerin you find in many natural and curly hair products and extremely humid or dry climates.

Here are a few common occlusives (you can read more about these occlusives in the section "Oils," later in the chapter):

» Coconut oil

» Grapeseed oil

» Castor oil

Oils versus butters

Which product is better — an oil or a butter? The answer depends on your hair goals and your hair texture. Oils tend to be lighter and work best for thinner strands, but butters — which are heavier and have bigger moisture molecules — work best on 3c to 4c hair. (For a rundown on different hair textures, head back to Chapter 3.) The butter actually penetrates the shaft and weighs down thinner strands, like 2a to 3b tresses.

Butters provide a protective barrier and can better stick to thick strands than oils can. If you have fine strands, such as 2a to 3b, lighter oils that don't weigh hair down are best.

Whichever route you choose, oils or butter, you need to seal the hair to protect it and prepare it for daily styling. Using oil or butter helps reduce frizz, saves time on detangling, increases length retention, and softens the hair.

Investigating Amazing Ingredients That Double as Supplements

Many ingredients that are great for topical hair care products are also safe and good for ingesting. The following sections give you a quick rundown of ingredients that enhance your hair products and keep your hair and scalp healthy. You can also work them into your vitamin and supplement routine.

Vitamin E

You probably know vitamin E for its antioxidant properties. For years, the skin industry has used vitamin E to combat aging, inflammation, and sun damage. Lately, in-the-know hair mavens have adopted vitamin E as a cure-all to turn frizzy, damaged, unruly hair into shiny, luscious strands fit for a highly liked Instagram image. Vitamin E can improve your overall scalp and hair health because it helps reduce oxidative stress (when you don't produce enough antioxidants to fight off free radicals), which often leads to hair loss.

Biotin

Biotin is a nutrient that helps to protect and rebuild your hair when excessive styling and harsh environmental conditions damage it. Biotin develops amino acids that structure the keratin protein, and it also invigorates the development of hair strands. If you want to consume biotin, you can find it naturally in several foods such as milk, eggs, and bananas.

TIP

Biotin is one of the most effective hair growth supplements because it stimulates keratin production and increases the rate of follicle production. I suggest taking at least 2,500 micrograms (mcg) per serving.

Vitamin B6

Vitamin B6 helps reduce the production of sebum that naturally comes from your scalp. When your production of sebum is in overdrive, you can end up with very oily skin and scalp, which causes your pores to clog. Vitamin B6 calms your *sebaceous glands* (the glands responsible for sebum production), allowing your follicles to grow from a healthy foundation. When you have balanced sebaceous glands, you can prevent sebum buildup at your scalp, which enables you to go a little longer between wash days during those lazy weeks.

WARNING

If you have dry hair, do not use vitamin B6, as you need as much oil as your hair will produce.

Vitamin B6 also enhances the circulation of oxygenated blood to the hair follicles and scalp. This blood flow considerably supports hair growth and hair strengthening.

Selenium

Selenium has several great benefits for your hair and scalp. Selenium contains antioxidant enzymes that can prevent your hair follicles from being damaged by sun rays, pollution, and other free radicals. Selenium can also help your body transform proteins to promote hair growth. Lastly, selenium is anti-inflammatory and kills dandruff-causing fungus. This is why you may see selenium as one of the top ingredients in a lot of treatments for dandruff and dry scalp.

Avoiding the "Bad" Ingredients

You definitely want to know which ingredients to look for (which I talk about in the preceding sections), but you also need to know which ingredients you might want to steer clear of. A lot of mass-produced hair products include substances that don't help your hair. Some of these products include ingredients that even damage your hair. Now here's the rub: All of these ingredients are bad in a way, but some are also kind of necessary evils.

WARNING

Although some products still include these ingredients, the companies that manufacturing them use higher-quality versions so that they can market their products as "sulfate-free" (or free of whatever the ingredient may be).

The other caveat to this section: These ingredients affect different people differently. Some folks might have an allergic reaction, but others don't. Be informed and make decisions that are right for you and your hair.

The healthier products often cost more because they don't have cheap additives, but having healthy hair makes the price worth it. After all, why go through a book about taking care of your hair, only to have your hair care hard work undone by these unsavory characters?

Although I also discuss other ingredients in the following sections, if you have curls or natural hair, it's most important to avoid sulfates, parabens, and silicones.

Sulfates

Okay, so sulfates are supposed to be the main cleaning agents in shampoo. And yes, sulfates strip away dirt and oil, but — hold onto your fedora — they also typically tend to strip your hair of all of its lovely natural oils! As you can probably surmise, when your hair loses its natural oils, it ultimately dries out and breaks. And the thing is, sulfates have been a key ingredient in shampoo forever. So if you've ever wondered why you keep washing and conditioning, but your hair is still as dry as the desert in July, chances are sulfates are part of the problem.

Even before natural hair re-emerged as a fashion statement around 2007 and 2008, sulfates were considered highly controversial; and as a result, several hair care manufacturers have developed new sulfate-based formulations that don't dry your hair. While more people catch onto the harm that sulfates can do, the demand for sulfate-free shampoos and other products is on the rise.

So why haven't sulfates totally gone away? Well, sulfates make your soap sudsy, and most people think their hair isn't clean unless they see suds. The truth is, you can get your hair just as clean without sulfates and suds. I'll admit, even I like the suds *(shrug)*, but we're all better off giving them up. To start cutting the cord, just check ingredient lists for any ingredient with the word *sulfate* in it. If you see sulfate, pass on that product.

Parabens

Parabens are preservatives used to give products a longer shelf life, but these chemicals can dry out your hair and cause frizz. Plus, parabens can enter your body through your scalp, disrupting your hormones and causing other serious medical issues. Similar to sulfates, keep your eyes out for the word *paraben* in the ingredients list. Just a heads up: You might find it tacked onto another word, looking something like *methylparaben,* so don't let it trick you.

Silicones

Silicones are man-made ingredients that manufacturers use to give hair the moisturized feeling of slippage. Notice that I say *feeling.* Silicones don't actually hydrate your hair. The silicone sits on the hair strands, which — when used regularly — can weigh down the hair because of excessive build up (flip back to Chapter 4 for guidance on removing buildup).

Alcohols

In general, alcohol dries things out, and the key to beautiful bouncing curls is moisture. So staying away from hair products that contain alcohol makes sense, right? Well, not all alcohols are created equal.

TECHNICAL
STUFF

Beware of short-chain alcohols, which have a shorter molecular structure than long-chain alcohols, allowing them to evaporate quickly. But this also dries hair out and causes it to be brittle. Here are a few examples:

>> Alcohol denat

>> Aminomethyl propanol

>> Ethanol

>> Isopropyl alcohol

>> Propyl alcohol

>> SD alcohol; SD alcohol 40

Stay away from the alcohols in the preceding list as much as possible. These alcohols can ultimately damage your hair cuticle, resulting in dry and frizzy hair. Now that I've told you the general rule, do you know what I'm going to tell you next? Yep, the exception to the rule!

TIP

Truthfully, if you need to cut down drying time or make applying styling products on your hair easier, alcohols can help — but only in small quantities. And not all the time.

FATTY ALCOHOLS

Unlike short-chain alcohols, which I talk about in the section "Alcohols," in this chapter, fatty alcohols don't dry your hair an excessive amount. They have a higher carbon content, which makes products feel oilier. Manufacturers often use fatty alcohols in their emollients (see the section "Emollients," in this chapter, for more on that hair care must-have). Fatty alcohols help make your hair feel smoother by making the cuticle lie flat. But like anything, if you use fatty acids in excess, you can cause problems such as stringy and greasy hair from the fatty acids combining with your hair's natural sebum. Here are some common fatty alcohols you might find in hair products:

- **Behenyl alcohol:** Synthetic or plant derived; a thickening agent used primarily to thicken creamy products and to soften and smooth hair

- **Benzyl alcohol:** A preservative or stabilizing agent derived from fruit; unlikely to impact hair texture in any way

- **Cetearyl alcohol:** A mix of alcohols that forms a white waxy solid and serves as an emollient or softener; most often found in cream-based products

- **Cetyl alcohol:** A waxy solid derived from plants or animals; used in creams and lotions to add viscosity and prevent oils and liquids from separating

- **Lauryl alcohol:** An organic compound produced industrially from palm kernel oil or coconut oil; keeps all the ingredients bound together for full and even application

- **Myristyl alcohol:** A lighter-weight fatty alcohol that functions as a thickener and emulsion stabilizer; keeps the liquids from separating while also softening the hair

- **Propylene glycol:** An additive that helps to preserve or stabilize products; often also used as a humectant (discussed in the section "Humectants," in this chapter)

- **Stearyl alcohol:** Vegetable derived; an emollient used to thicken and emulsify a variety of cosmetic products

Fragrance

Many natural ingredients have their own smell (for example, coconut oil, mint, and eucalyptus). I'm not talking about those fragrances in this section. What I *am* warning you about are synthetic fragrances and scents that manufacturers use to get your attention and make their products more appealing to you. Companies do a lot of research to find the most popular smells to appeal to your senses. But honestly, in hair care, fragrance is totally non-essential, and it can even be damaging.

The primary ingredient of most fragrance is alcohol, and you know what that means: Unless you want dried out hair, run away! (See the section "Alcohols," earlier in this chapter, for the rundown of these frizz-creators.)

However, some brands have gone so far as to create hair fragrances that you spritz on your hair rather than your body. I don't want to tell you what to do with your life, so I'll just say — maybe not.

TIP

But if you love all things that smell good, don't feel shame. Try essential oils, which provide a great alternative to synthetic fragrances. Try adding a few drops of citrus, lavender, eucalyptus, tea tree, or floral oils to your water bottle and mist your hair. Or add essential oils into your hair oil when you use it as a sealant!

Choosing Products That Work Best for Your Hair

It's time to stock your shelves! The following sections tell you all about which types of products you can buy to address your personal hair care needs and characteristics. From shampoos to mousse, and from edge control to butters, I get you all set up.

Shampoos

Shampoos are the main product you use to cleanse your hair, and there are different kinds of shampoos you can use to achieve different levels of cleansing. Although you may see more than this when you shop in a retail store or online, the four main categories should know about and use are:

>> Regular/normal shampoo

>> Clarifying shampoo

>> Moisturizing/hydrating shampoo

>> Dry shampoo

You may need to use only one kind of shampoo, or you may find yourself using all four.

Regular/normal

Regular or normal shampoo simply cleans your hair and scalp from excess oils and buildup. They don't address any specific hair needs or treatments, other than cleansing your hair with straightforward ingredients without stripping your scalp's natural oils. When you shop for regular shampoo, some of the best ingredients to look for include plant oils, fruit extracts, and aloe vera. These ingredients clean natural and curly hair without drying it out too much, as well as preserve your curl pattern.

Clarifying

When you want to clean your hair more deeply, use a clarifying shampoo. It thoroughly removes excess product buildup and residue from your hair and scalp because it contains a *chelating agent,* which is a chemical compound that binds to iron and other metallic material, dissolves it, and then makes it easy for the water to rinse away.

TECHNICAL STUFF

When you are shopping for clarifying shampoos, pass up any that have harsh sulfates, and keep your eye out for chelating agents in the ingredient list. Tetrasodium EDTA and tetrahydroxypropyl ethylenediamine is the most common chelating agent.

If you use products regularly, you should have a clarifying shampoo in your hair care regimen. When you use clarifying shampoo, it cleans your hair so deeply that it helps your conditioners, masks, and treatments penetrate better.

After using a clarifying shampoo, your hair will feel squeaky clean because it's been stripped of its natural oils and may feel hard to touch. Follow your clarifying shampoo up with a moisturizing shampoo or your favorite conditioner to replenish the moisture and soften the hair shaft (more on that in Chapter 4).

Moisturizing/hydrating

Moisturization and hydration is commonly used interchangeably when it comes to natural and curly hair, but there is a difference that is important to know when you're shampoo shopping. Ingredients in hydrating shampoos attract or add water to the hair, increasing moisture content in your strands. Moisturizing shampoos prevent moisture loss by locking or sealing water in the hair.

Let's say your hair is dry, and you're looking for a shampoo to help you put moisture back into your actual hair strands. You should select a hydrating shampoo. If your hair isn't dry, but you want to keep the level of moisture it has in it safe, use a moisturizing shampoo to lock that moisture in. You can also use both: a hydrating shampoo first to put water into the hair, and then a moisturizing shampoo second to lock that new water in.

Both of these types of shampoos contain detergent (or cleansing agents) to rid your hair and scalp of dirt, sebum and product buildup, and odor.

Dry

Dry shampoo is not typically a go-to for the natural and curly hair community because they are mostly marketed and seen being used by people with Type 1 hair, but since most natural and curly hair types don't require multiple washes throughout the week, dry, shampoos can be great to add to your weekly routine because it absorbs the oils, dirt, and grease from your hair and scalp without using water (it's an aerosol spray product).

You can use dry shampoo to freshen up your hair after working out, to extend a blowout style, or prolong the time between wash days.

I always have dry shampoo in my kit while on set just in case a client doesn't arrive with freshly cleaned hair, as it's my pro solution to help several-days-old hair look fresh.

TIP

When testing out dry shampoos, look for a virtually invisible one so you won't be left with a chalky cast. You might have to try a few different dry shampoos to find the one that is invisible on your specific hair.

Detangling conditioners

You should definitely have a detangling conditioner in your collection. As the name suggests, it helps you detangle your hair because it contains a lot of *slip* (or lubrication), which makes it easy for your wide-tooth comb to glide through your hair with little to no friction, letting you comb out and untangle your hair easily.

Detangling conditioners are so lubricating because they don't sink into the hair shaft. Instead, they sit on the surface and coat the hair shaft, which makes your hair easier to detangle because it smooths the cuticle layer.

Select a detangling conditioner with these ingredients that provide the most slip:

>> Plant oils like olive or coconut

>> Butters like shea or cocoa

>> Glycerin (natural or organic)

>> Silicones (Make sure you read the section, "Avoiding the 'Bad' Ingredients" in this chapter before choosing a product with silicones.)

A NOTE ABOUT CO-WASHES

The *co* in "co-wash" is short for "conditioner." Simply put, co-washing is when you use conditioner to cleanse your hair instead of a shampoo because you want the extra hydration and moisture that the conditioner offers. Although there are products out there specifically marketed for co-washing, you really don't need to buy them. Your favorite conditioner contains cleansing agents in it and can clean your hair while protecting the moisture. For more info on co-washing, turn back to Chapter 4.

Twisting creams

When you want to define and elongate your curls, add twisting cream to your hair product collection. Twisting creams provide natural shine and hold when you apply them to your damp hair. When you apply a little twisting cream to your twist out, wash-and-go's, or diffused or air-dried styles, you can preserve your curl pattern and moisture.

When you are shopping for one, look for a cream that is lightweight, non-sticky, non-flaky, and non-greasy. Select a cream that has water as one of the first three ingredients and contains ingredients like glycerin, aloe vera, and shea butter.

Gels, mousses, and curl definers

No matter your hair type, to give your style a nice finished, polished look that keeps your curls rockin' without frizzing up, use gels, mousses, or curl definers. They all help your hair to stay in place without gluing your strands down or letting them dry out. But each of these products have slightly different features, and you may have to try different products and brands to find what works for you.

- » **Gels:** Reduce friction, minimize frizz, hold your hairstyles in place, lay and smooth your hairline/edges, and keep your curls defined without making them look or feel crunchy. Look for gels that are labeled "flake-free" and don't have alcohol listed in the ingredients.

- » **Mousses:** Also help with hold and minimizing frizz. Similar to gels, mousses reduce friction making it easier to style your hair. But unlike gels, mousses are great for adding volume to finer hair textures as they work to plump up the hair shaft, creating the illusion of thicker strands. Look for a mousse that doesn't weigh your hair down and is also alcohol free.

- » **Curl definers:** Help you sculpt define and smooth your curls. To add defini-tion to your curls using a curl definer, apply some with your hands to your wet hair from root to ends, making sure it's evenly distributed, and then scrunch to form your curl pattern, and dry as desired (whether by using a dryer or air-drying). When shopping for curl definers, look for ingredients like coconut oil, Jardin oil, green tea extract, jojoba oil, and olive oil.

TIP

Now you know me; I don't recommend many specific products, but I just have to share this one with you. That's how good it is. My favorite curl cream for wash-and-gos is the Coconut Curling Cream from Cantu (see Figure 7-1). It conditions your hair, plus adds definition and make your curls soft and manageable. I especially love that it's made with pure shea butter and no harsh ingredients. It even won an award in 2013, when it was named Best of the Best by NaturallyCurly.com! (PDC Brands pays me an influencer fee to promote this Cantu product.)

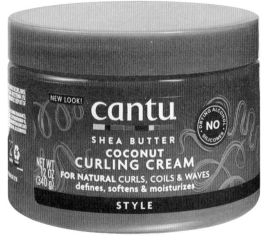

FIGURE 7-1:
Coconut Curling
Cream from
Cantu.

Courtesy of Cantu

Edge control

Edge control, a gel-like product that's much thicker and less pliable than most products used on natural hair, can help you tame or style your hairline or baby hair like nothing else. Choose a formula based on your hair texture so that your hair ends up neither greasy nor sticky. For finer strands, you can use an edge control that's more fluid in texture — almost like a pomade or something that you can use for flyaways, like serums. For thicker and coarse strands, go for a thick but non-greasy tamer that's also heat resistant so that your edges stay laid even in the summer.

Conditioners and hair masks

Moisture is fundamental for keeping your luscious kinks and curls in the best shape possible. (If you don't believe me, flip to the section "Focusing on the Holy

Grail of Hair Care," earlier in this chapter.) Conditioner makes each strand of hair smooth and reduces frizz by helping the cuticle layer lay down flat (for a refresher on the conditioner and hair mask 411, turn back to Chapter 4). But I know you might find selecting the right conditioner or mask for your hair confusing. You can find so many different variations of conditioner out there that do different things to and for your hair. Allow me to break it down for you:

>> **Regular conditioners:** Typically used after you shampoo for 5 to 10 minutes, you might hear these called *surface conditioners* because they soften your hair only at the surface level. If your hair is a tad dry but the overall condition of your hair is good, you can use regular conditioners for maintenance every time you shampoo.

>> **Deep conditioners:** Intended to stay on your hair for 15 to 30 minutes, deep conditioners are typically much thicker in appearance than surface conditioners. They soften deeper into the core of the hair strand and keep your hair conditioned for a much longer time than a surface conditioner. In general, you can deep condition two to four times per month. Deep conditioners can really help you out if you experience a little more dryness and shedding than normal, whether it's occasional or chronic.

>> **Hair masks:** Made to strengthen and repair your hair. Leave hair masks on for 20 to 30 minutes. They're highly concentrated with additives that can help revitalize your hair. You can use hair masks about once or twice per week, in place of your surface conditioner. If your hair is colored, has weakened elasticity from excessive tension, or has some heat damage, or you're transitioning from a relaxer, a good mask can help you repair and restore your hair's integrity.

>> **Leave-in conditioners:** You can use leave-in conditioners as an additional conditioner to give you some extra moisture and protection. Look for something lightweight that also offers heat protection from both UV rays and styling tools. You can find leave-ins available in two different forms: liquid spray for a light, weightless feel, and product with a milky to creamy texture that you rub into the hair. If you have wavy to loose curls, go for spray-on, but tighter curls should use creamier leave-ins to help the curls retain moisture (which gives better curl definition and separation).

REMEMBER

All products are made differently, so make sure to always follow the manufacturer's instructions.

Oils

When it's time for your hot oil treatment (flip back to Chapter 4 for more on how to do them and how often), you can either buy a premade version from the store, or you can make your own.

You can use many different oils for hair treatments. When figuring out which one to select, it comes down to what your hair needs. Do you need to hydrate it? Moisturize it? Both? You can choose to use one oil or a combination of several oils.

Lightweight oils act more like humectants (which I talk about in the section "Humectants," earlier in this chapter) and can penetrate your actual hair shaft. Use these oils if your hair is very dry or damaged and you're just beginning your hot-oil journey. Here are a few options:

>> **Amla oil:** A great choice if you have an oily scalp but dry hair. It strengthens and conditions all parts of your hair, down to the root.

>> **Avocado oil:** Fights frizz like no other. If you need some radiant shine and extra growth, go with this oil.

>> **Coconut oil:** The best option if you have some pesky dandruff you want to ditch. Coconut oil also strengthens your hair because of the proteins it contains that bind to your shaft.

>> **Cetrimonium chloride:** A great option for battling static and frizz, plus has detangling properties.

>> **Grapeseed oil:** Excellent if you have brittle hair or need to protect it against heat or thermal styling. This oil can also help you treat and prevent dandruff.

>> **Olive oil:** Olive oil can soften your hair up and add some shine to boot. Fatty oils act more like emollients and occlusives, moisturizing from the outside to lock in moisture. Flip back to the sections "Emollients" and "Occlusives (a.k.a. sealants)," earlier in this chapter, to get the details on these types of products. These oils allow you to maintain your lovely locs, after you give yourself any number of treatments.

>> **Castor oil:** Use this oil if you're in cold weather or want to get rid of buildup. Castor oil is also anti-inflammatory and promotes hair growth thanks to nutrients such as vitamin A, Omega 6 and other fatty acids, and proteins.

The two types of castor oil are yellow, which is cold-pressed, and Jamaican black castor oil (JBCO), which uses roasted castor beans. JBCO has a higher pH and is more alkaline than yellow castor oil, so you can use JBCO as a clarifying agent.

>> **Jojoba oil:** Rich in vitamins and minerals that nourish your hair, including vitamin C, B vitamins, vitamin E, copper, and zinc. Make this oil your go-to if you have dry hair or scalp because it's so similar to the natural sebum your hair follicles produce that sometimes your body can't even tell the difference. It also has antibacterial properties.

>> **Grapeseed oil:** Excellent if you have brittle hair or need to protect it against heat or thermal styling because it has a lot of vitamin E and fatty acids. It can also help you treat and prevent dandruff.

After you know which oils can help you manage your hair, you can shop with confidence and grab some perfect premade options off the shelf. Or if you're feeling bold, you can try your hand at making your own oil-based hair product.

TIP

The lists in this section can get you started, but you can find more oils out there beyond the options I talk about. So don't be afraid to do additional research, ask your friends, and experiment to see what works for you.

Butters

When you need a moisture-lock product that's thicker than your hair, go with butters. Butters make sure that all your hair's hard-earned hydration doesn't vanish in a flash. Butters are best for coarse and thick hair, but you can still use them if you have fine or thin hair; just start with small amounts. Here's a list of some butters to try:

>> **Shea butter:** The most perfect butter to help soothe your dry hair. It smooths out the cuticle, or surface, of your hair because it contains a lot of fatty acids.

>> **Cocoa butter:** If you have fine or thin hair, cocoa butter can help you maintain long-term hydration and supports healthy oil production to help prevent breakage.

>> **Mango butter:** Keeps your hair moisturized, but with bounce and fluff. Mango butter also provides excellent UV protection. It's lighter than shea butter, so it doesn't leave as much buildup. And it's the perfect alternative if you're allergic to shea butter.

Heat protectants

Heat protectants create a barrier between your hair and direct heat so the heat doesn't damage your hair. Apply a heat protectant before you use any hot tool (see more on those tools in Chapter 8). The protectant helps you prevent frizz by locking in moisture by sealing your cuticle. When selecting a heat protectant

>> Choose a protectant that indicates on the label that it provides maximum heat protection.

>> Read the ingredient list to make sure keratin is one of the first ingredients listed. Keratin adds protein to your hair, which increases its strength.

>> Read the ingredient list to make sure the protectant contains organic silicones such as cyclomethicone and dimenthicone, which will coat and protect your hair from drying out.

Turning Your Kitchen into a DIY Product Treasure Trove

If you want to avoid wading through store-bought hair care products, you can always make your own. If you like to stay away from chemicals but are open to adventure, you might want to go the DIY route. In today's world, you have access to all the information you need to craft your own shampoo, conditioner, hair masks, and other products. Unfortunately, I don't have the space to detail all of the different recipes for all of the different products you could potentially make. But a quick Internet search can give you all the ideas you could ever want. Look for sites that are written by professionals in the natural hair care world.

Here and now, I can give you a quick list of items you probably already have in your house that you can put to work immediately on their own to hydrate and moisturize your lustrous locs.

Throughout this chapter, I mention different natural ingredients that you can find at home to use on your hair as single-item care and treatment. I don't repeat any of them in this list, but make no mistake: These ingredients can improve your DIY game, so go back through and search them out if you need to!

Without further ado, here's a list of time-tested, tried-and-true DIY hair care ideas:

>> **Honey:** A great natural humectant, you can use honey with water or oil, or incorporate it into another natural hair treatment. Honey can promote cell growth, help your hair retain moisture, and restore nutrients to your hair and scalp. It may even help alleviate any inflammatory skin conditions you're dealing with when you combine it with other therapies. You can also use honey to treat dandruff, clean hair follicles, increase shine, and more.

The simplest way to use honey on your hair is to combine 1 cup of honey and ¼ cup olive oil, then massage the mixture into your scalp and hair. Let it sit for 1 to 2 hours. Rinse, then shampoo and condition like you would normally. However, if you want to be fancy, you can find all sorts of recipes online that teach you how to make your own honey hair mask!

>> **Aloe:** Has innumerable health benefits, including many for natural hair. Aloe vera contains vitamins A, B12, C, and E, which are said to promote hair growth, and its natural enzymes aid in hair retention (which means less shedding) and soothe dry and itchy scalp (which lead to dandruff). Because of aloe's viscosity, it serves as an excellent protective layer on the hair.

Apply aloe vera gel into your scalp and gently massage it in. You can also apply it to your strands. Make sure to leave the aloe gel or juice on for at least 2 hours before rinsing or washing your hair. You should notice an improvement in the condition of your scalp and hair in about 2 to 3 months.

>> **Rice:** Full of amino acids, B vitamins, and antioxidants, you can use rice to detangle your hair and make it shiny and smooth. Well, technically, you make rice water.

Combine ½ cup of rinsed uncooked rice with 2 to 3 cups of water. Let the rice soak for about a half-hour, and then strain it. After you shampoo and rinse your hair, pour the rice water on your hair, massage it into your hair and scalp, and let it sit for about 20 minutes. After that, rinse with warm water.

>> **Flaxseed gel:** A secret-sauce hair mask for getting your curls to clump without frizz. Also, this gel fortifies the follicles, leading to moisturized hair that grows faster and longer.

To make your own flaxseed gel, simmer 4 tablespoons of flaxseeds in 2 cups of water for 2 to 3 minutes over medium heat. Stir and strain the flaxseeds through a cheesecloth. Cool for up to 2 hours. You can use this gel on clean and conditioned hair by massaging a small amount onto your hair. Leave it to sit for 15 minutes, then rinse and shampoo and condition normally.

>> **Apple cider vinegar (ACV):** Rich in vitamins B and C, ACV also contains alpha-hydroxy acid, which *exfoliates* the scalp (removes dead skin cells) and serves as an anti-inflammatory to help prevent dandruff.

On wash day, use it as a scalp cleanser (find more about cleansing your scalp in Chapter 4).

>> **Tea tree oil:** An antibacterial and antifungal, tea tree oil helps soothe dry itchy scalps (see Chapter 4 for application tips).

>> **Peppermint oil:** An antimicrobial and anti-inflammatory, peppermint oil penetrates the hair follicle and aids in blood circulation, which can help with hair growth.

You can get the most out of peppermint oil as a pre-shampoo on wash day because it removes buildup, reduces inflammation, and gives the hair extra moisture (for more details about how to apply it, flip back to Chapter 4).

IN THIS CHAPTER

» Discovering the difference
between detangling and drying
brushes

» Using the right combs

» Using hot tools in safe ways

Chapter **8**

Selecting and Mastering Tools

B ecause of how delicate your natural curls are, you must handle them with gentle care to maintain their curl pattern and overall health. In addition to careful handling (which I talk about in Chapter 6) and using the perfect products (check out Chapter 7), selecting and mastering the right styling tools for your hair sets you up for success. These tools can make your wash day more efficient and help you create and maintain your styles more easily.

Back in the day, natural hair care tools were practically absent from beauty-supply and drugstores. Or at least, no one specifically marketed them for curly textures. Over the past 15 years, brands have expanded their natural hair tool selections and advertising to directly cater to people who have wavy, coily, and kinky textures. As the natural hair community continues to thrive, you can expect brands to develop more products and tools to help you style and maintain the health of your hair.

This chapter hopefully saves you the guesswork in selecting and using the right tools. No matter the various hair types and textures — whether your curl pattern is 2a wavy or 4c coily — all people who have natural or curly hair need the same basic tools. However, over time and with some experimentation, you can find tools that fit your unique styling routine. So get prepared to transform your bathroom into a mini natural hair salon!

Brushes

Brushes don't come with descriptive labels in the same way that your shampoo and conditioner bottles do, so how do you know where to start? You have so many brushes to choose from on the market, and they all have different jobs and features. Some are great with dry hair, but not wet hair. Some help you with styling, and you can use others to detangle. Some — but not all — can be both!

You may find your brush choices overwhelming, but I'm here to help. Because you have so much versatility with styling your natural hair, you need a variety of brushes in your arsenal. In the following sections, I give you a few options, how they function, and what to look for when selecting brushes.

A brush to detangle, a brush to dry

To take the best care of your (or your loved one's) natural and curly hair, have one brush that you use to detangle your hair and one that you use to dry your hair. You've probably seen different brushes marketed as detangling brushes and others marketed as drying brushes. These categories aren't just a marketing ploy; you actually need a separate brush for each task. Although you can use your drying brush for detangling, don't use your detangling brush for drying because detangling brushes are not made to stand up to the heat you use while drying your hair. You can use drying brushes to stretch out your curls while drying them with heat.

WARNING

Detangling brushes can't handle direct heat. Never use them while drying your hair because direct heat causes them to deteriorate.

Like the name suggests, you use *detangling brushes* on wet hair to remove tangles and knots. Although you don't need to use them every day, detangling brushes see a lot of action on wash day, so you want to make sure to get one that you like and that holds up to a lot of use. When selecting a detangling brush, look for several key features

>> Firm bristles that maintain their shape during detangling.

>> Cone-shaped, smooth plastic bristles (this bristle shape helps the brush gently separate your strands of hair).

>> A sturdy handle gives you the stability you need to brush and dry your hair efficiently and thoroughly.

You have some great options to choose from out there.

Felicia Leatherwood detailer brush

My personal go-to — and a favorite among hairstylists, in general — is the Felicia Leatherwood detangler brush (see Figure 8-1). It has the best design for detangling your hair smoothly. It has nine individual flexible rows of strong, smooth bristles. Basically, it's like you have nine wide-tooth combs positioned side-by-side, all connected to one handle that forms a brush. This design helps you gently detangle knots in half the time of other detangling brushes, and you can also use it to evenly spread product and create perfectly defined curls. This brush works amazingly well to detangle high density, 4c hair without snagging because of its unique design, but you can use it on all textures and types.

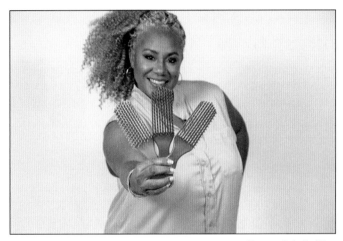

Photography by Teal Moss

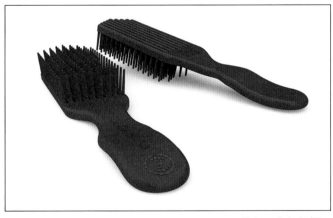

FIGURE 8-1:
The Felicia Leatherwood detangler brush's design and function makes detangling a breeze.

Photography by Teal Moss

Paddle brush

If you want a brush that you can use for both detangling and drying, get a *paddle brush.* As the name suggests, they look like a paddle — wide and flat. Paddle brushes work best for fine to medium hair types. They have flexible, cushioned bases, and their bristles are a little thinner than regular detangling brushes. You can use them for working out knots and under heat when doing blowouts.

Paddle brushes begin to melt after repeated exposure to heat, so you have to replace them often.

I like to use paddle brushes after shampooing, after I saturate the hair with rinse-out conditioner. These brushes really help you spread the conditioner evenly throughout the hair, from root to tip, and they also help remove any tangles that you create while shampooing.

When shopping for a paddle brush (see Figure 8-2), look for strong rubber handles and bristles that have a tiny bulb at the end. The handles are sturdy enough for detangling, and the bulbs aid in massaging your scalp.

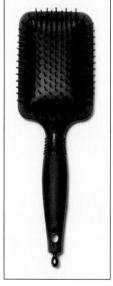

FIGURE 8-2: When selecting a paddle brush, look for strong rubber handles and tiny bulbs.

Photography by Wardell Malloy with crowdMGMT

If you want a brush that detangles and that definitely holds up to heat, try a Denman brush (see Figure 8-3). It has an extremely durable and sleek design that makes it great for detangling, defining, and even blowing out your natural curls because it can stand up to heat. In fact, this is the only brush I use for drying!

The natural hair community loves the Denman brush because it's long-lasting, it stands up to heat, and it's comfortable in your hand and on your head. I particularly love them for blow drying because they are so strong.

Its rubber base and smooth, plastic pins (bristles) glide through your curls and ensure beautiful curl definition without damage and frizz. The rubber base, combined with the closeness of the pins, grips the hair nice and taut while you blow it out straight. Denman brushes are delicate enough to create wash-and-go styles and sturdy enough for your occasional silky blowouts. They can also help you with shingling. Flip back to Chapter 4 for how-tos on that.

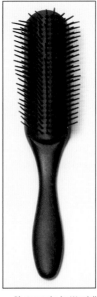

FIGURE 8-3: Another example of a paddle brush.

Photography by Wardell Malloy with crowdMGMT

Boar bristle brushes

A good boar bristle brush is one of the most important tools to have in your hair care collection for achieving the killer style you want. Although some boar bristle brushes are soft, which are perfect for younger children and folks who are tender-headed, naturalistas more commonly use stiff bristle brushes. Do you ever wonder how people get those amazing, shiny, smooth looks without a smidge of frizz? They use stiff bristle brushes.

When you want to rock a smooth ponytail (a *snatchback*), stiff bristle brushes get the job done. They come in different shapes and sizes — even small enough for your hairline, making it easy to tame your edges and style baby hairs (the wispy hair around your hairline)! With the right styling product and a stiff bristle brush, you can make your hair completely frizz free.

REMEMBER

Boar bristle brushes are like toothbrushes; some people prefer soft and some people prefer stiff. If you want a polished look and can withstand the force of a stiff brush, use it. If you have a lighter job or don't want as much force on your scalp, use a soft brush.

TIP

You can use boar bristle brushes on all hair types and textures, but if you have fine and fragile hair, search for a soft bristle brush.

These brushes help

>> Stimulate blood circulation in the scalp, which promotes hair growth.

>> Distribute your natural oils from the roots to the ends.

>> Detangle on wash day because they loosen dirt and debris.

REMEMBER

When shopping for a bristle brush, check to confirm that it's made from pure boar bristles (see Figure 8-4). Although you can find bristle brushes made of all materials, bristle brushes that use actual boar bristles are the optimum. Because boar hair is similar to human hair, they are gentler on the hair shaft and can move through strands better than nylon brushes that get snagged.

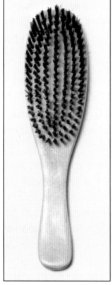

FIGURE 8-4:
Boar bristle brushes are the industry standard for perfectly sleek styles.

Photography by Wardell Malloy with crowdMGMT

Getting to Know Your Combs

You can use several different types of combs while you're styling and caring for your natural hair. Depending on how tender or sensitive your scalp feels, combing natural hair can be a little painful. But if you use the right tools and the right techniques, you can comb without pain or breakage.

Before I get into the combs, here are a few of my favorite tips for mastering them.

Do:

>> Use a comb on dry natural hair only when you have a silky blowout or an afro (technically you would use a pick on an afro).

>> Work in small sections to detangle your hair.

>> Start from the ends of your hair and work your way up to your scalp.

Don't:

>> (Almost) never comb natural curly hair while it's dry. Spray some water and leave-in conditioner on your curls first. Then, you can comb.

>> Never use a fine-tooth comb for detangling.

To keep your natural hair looking fine, have a few different types of combs in your tool collection. The following sections give you a rundown of how these different combs function and what to look for when purchasing them.

Fine-tooth combs

You can identify *fine-tooth combs* by their narrow, close set of teeth (see Figure 8-5). They grab your hair tightly and get it perfectly straight and settled into place. Fine-tooth combs are great for

>> Combing through silky blowouts.

>> Creating a clean, polished ponytail.

>> Removing dry skin and buildup off the scalp before shampooing on wash day. Focus on only the scalp area and avoid pulling the comb through your curls, which can cause snagging and breakage.

When purchasing a fine-tooth comb, look for one made from a strong, heat-resistant hard rubber or carbon material. These combs are a little more expensive than the flimsy, plastic combs, but they're salon-quality and built to last, which makes your styling experience positive.

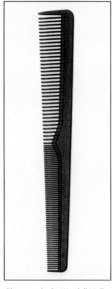

FIGURE 8-5:
A fine-tooth comb.

Photography by Wardell Malloy with crowdMGMT

Wide-tooth combs

The natural hair community embraces wide-tooth combs because they detangle well. *Wide-tooth combs* have thick, wide-set teeth that allow a lot of hair to glide through easily (see Figure 8-6). Use this comb to minimize breakage when you need to comb your knots out during detangling or to separate your hair.

When purchasing a wide-tooth comb, look for combs made of wood or hard rubber because they are durable, or cellulose acetate, which has anti-static properties.

My absolute favorite is the 9-inch Hercules Sägemann Magic Star Comb made of 100% natural rubber. It's handmade and very durable, feels extremely comfortable in your hand, and always gets the job done.

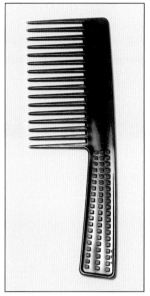

FIGURE 8-6:
A wide-tooth
comb.

Photography by Wardell Malloy
with crowdMGMT

Rat tail combs

Rat tail combs have a comb on one end and a sectioning point on the other. The sectioning point kind of looks like a straight rat's tail (that's how it got its name). These features elevate your styles by helping you create straight, clean partings. Rat tail combs help you part and/or section your hair. You can use a regular comb if you like, but you can't part your sections as cleanly (straight and evenly) as you can with a rat tail comb.

Also, rat tail combs are excellent for styling comb-twists (for more on creating them, flip back to Chapter 5).

Although I don't recommend combing out knots by using rat tail combs, these combs can help you detangle tight, stubborn knots. When you find a knot, push the tail end (or point) of the comb into the knot and gently move the comb end around to loosen the knot.

If you're shopping for a rat tail comb, look for the same materials that you would with a fine-tooth or wide-tooth comb (see the preceding sections), plus a stainless-steel sectioning point (see Figure 8-7). You can find rat tail combs with points that are made of whatever material the comb is (like wood or plastic), but I prefer steel because it's thin, strong, and gives clean parts. Most rat tail combs have fine teeth, but you also can find rat tail combs that have wide teeth, if you prefer. Fine teeth help you grab the hair and keep it close for smooth styling, while wide teeth provide the ability to detangle.

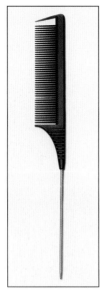

FIGURE 8-7:
A rat tail comb.

Hair picks

If you want big, voluminous curls, add a hair pick to your tool collection. Hair picks are square-shaped, similar to a painter's brush, and have long, semi-wide, stiff teeth that can help you style and detangle your hair. Plastic picks are gentle on your curls, making them perfect for all hair types.

You can master using picks in no time. It's easy to use them in your styling, which makes them a very useful tool. Use hair picks to fluff out an afro of any size. Or add fullness and volume to twist outs and wash-and-go's by using a pick right at the base of your style, near the scalp. Lift gently to create fullness without pulling the pick completely through your curls (see Figure 8-8).

When purchasing a hair pick, don't go cheap or thin. Spend a little extra time and money; choose a strong plastic pick so it doesn't break. Look for a pick that doesn't give a lot of flex and stands up to a little pressure if you try to push it.

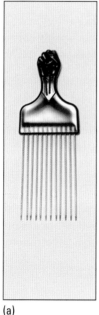

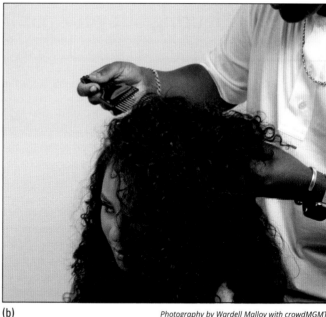

FIGURE 8-8:
Use a pick (a) to add volume to your hair (b). (a)   (b)

Applying Heat

Deciding whether to use heat (or hot) tools is always a major concern among naturals. If you're worried about giving your hair heat damage after using these tools, you're not alone. I totally get it! But here's the scoop: Heat damage happens when you don't have the right tools — or you use the tools incorrectly. When you use hot tools properly, you can set your hair, add texture, define curls, and safely straighten your hair for an occasional silky blowouts. The following sections tell you what to look for in different types of heat-styling tools.

REMEMBER

Some stylists think using any styling product before applying heat offers all the heat protection you need. Although I can see their point of view, I disagree. Heat protectant products are specifically designed to create a barrier between your hair strands and direct heat. Yes, styling products can provide some protection, but your hair can only benefit from more layers of protection. Heat protectants come in several different forms — serums, creams, sprays — and you can apply them very easily. So, don't skip this step. For more about picking the right heat protectant product, go back to Chapter 7.

Figuring out your flat iron

You can use a flat iron to straighten your natural hair. But because everyone has different hair types and textures, definitely don't go with a flat iron that has only an on-and-off switch. Look for a flat iron that has adjustable heat control settings. These heat settings give you control and allow you to select the proper setting to keep your unique curls safe. Medium to coarse hair can handle a higher heat setting, but use a lower heat setting for thin fine hair (go back to Chapter 6 for more on this). Flat irons typically have a heat range between 180 and 450 degrees Fahrenheit (82–232 degrees Celsius), so check out the dials before making your purchase.

Also look at the type of material that make up the plates. You can choose from the most common materials: ceramic, tourmaline, or titanium. They all have different claims and features. I could go on about the difference between these three plates for pages, but let me simplify it for you: The considerable difference between the materials involves the rate at and method by which they heat your hair. Here's a little bit about each material:

>> **Ceramic:** This plate heats up evenly and heats your hair from the inside out using infrared technology. I recommend ceramic plates for all hair textures, but especially fine to medium hair textures because the infrared technology allows the iron to use less heat by releasing negative ions, which lock moisture into your hair, creating a more gentle and less frizzing experience. Ceramic also glides through the hair easily and doesn't tug or pull. This is a good choice if you use flat irons infrequently.

>> **Tourmaline:** This material releases even more negative ions than ceramic, giving it more smoothing power. This makes it a good fit for thick or coarse hair. This plate straightens hair with less heat than ceramic or titanium and helps lay the cuticle flat with its high ion count. Tourmaline plates constantly generate negative ions, even when turned off. This feature helps give optimal results with less heat and is great for all hair types.

>> **Titanium:** This plate is really best for professionals. It heats the surface of the hair shaft, and then the heat travels inward. Titanium plates heat up quickly (almost instantly) and stay consistently hot while you use your iron. Titanium plates produce more negative ions than tourmaline plates, which helps smooth your hair and prevent frizz. Titanium plates work well on all hair textures, but because they can maintain heat for a long time, they're more efficient with thick, coarse hair.

WARNING

Be aware that if you don't use them properly, they can cause heat damage because of how quickly and high they heat, which means that titanium plates are best fit for professionals or folks who have experience or confidence with heat styling.

TIP

If you travel, look for a flat iron (or any heat styling tool) that has dual voltage so that you can safely use it abroad. Otherwise, you practically burn it out as soon as you plug it into a foreign outlet. That goes for all your electric hair tools.

To master your flat iron, follow these steps to get very good at this basic best practice:

1. **Heat your flat iron to the desired temperature.**

2. **Apply a heat protectant to your hair.**

3. **Divide your hair into four sections.**

4. **From one section, separate out a smaller section, about 1 to 1½ inches wide.**

    If you want maximum straightness, the smaller the section, the better. If you make your section too thick and wide, the heat can't get all the way through. The top and bottom of the section might be flat, but the middle stays crinkly.

5. **Place your hair between the flat iron, close it, and hold.**

    Start at the top of your hair near the root.

6. **Place a comb in your hair just below the flat iron.**

    The comb acts as a guide for your hair.

7. **Slide the iron and comb down your hair at the same time.**

8. **Repeat Steps 4 through 7 for all of your hair, but no more than once. The goal is to get it done in one pass.**

Bringing up blow dryers

You need a good blow dryer, plus the right skills to create some of your favorite styles without damaging your hair. There is no doubt that the market is oversaturated with blow dryers. Here are some key features to look for when purchasing yours:

» Professional-level power (look for 1875 watts or more)

» Variable heat control (including a cool shot button, which is a button that turns the air cool, allowing you to set your curls)

» Ionic technology (it allows the dryer to shoot negative ions into the water droplets that are on the hair shaft, which causes them to break up and prevents them from soaking in and causing your hair to frizz)

» Comb, nozzle, and diffuser attachments

MAKING THE MOST OF YOUR HAIRDRYER

If you already have your dryer, here are a few of my favorite tips for getting the most out of it:

- **Dry before drying.** After you shampoo and condition your hair, use a t-shirt to absorb the extra water before you use your blow dryer (flip back to Chapter 4 for a refresher on that technique).

- **Diffuse a wash-and-go.** If you want to dry your wash-and-go, use the diffuser attachment and hold the dryer about 6 inches from your hair. Dry sections of your head until your roots are only slight damp.

- **Dry and straighten at the same time.** If you want to straighten your hair, apply a heat protectant first. Then, section your hair into small sections about an inch to inch and a half wide. Then, place your brush underneath a small section of your hair and the blow dryer on top. Then, gently press your blow dryer against your brush while you create a bit of tension. This tension helps to smooth out your curls.

>> Lightweight

>> Multiple speed settings

You have to do your own research to find the right dryer for you. Ask your friends and family what they like (and if you can try theirs). Also, read as many reviews online as possible. I have my personal favorites, of course, if you need a little more direction. Out of hundreds of dryers to choose from, only two have kept my attention over the last few years and are absolutely worth the investment. One has a beautiful, chic design and offers everything I look for in a conventional blow dryer. The other has a revolutionized way of drying the hair in half the time and is ideal for stretching curls without damaging them.

The Dyson Supersonic hairdryer is a work of art. When this dryer first hit the market, I just had to get my hands on one, and I was so thrilled it lived up to the hype I created in my mind. Aside from its unique design, this lightweight dryer is compact and powerful. This dryer has three speed settings, four heat settings, and a cold shot button that helps you set your hair while styling. It has intelligent heat control that protects your hair from heat damage. It also has ionic technology that dries your hair faster than most other blow dryers, which increases smoothness and shine while decreasing frizz and flyaways. It comes with five magnetic styling attachments, but I use three of them the most, which also tend to be the most common:

>> **Wide-tooth comb:** Great for blowing out curls; has robust teeth that help straighten the hair while it dries.

>> **Styling concentrator:** Also great for blowouts because it helps you focus airflow on one section while you use a blow-drying brush. The rest of your hair remains undisturbed.

>> **Diffuser:** Disperses air evenly around your curls, helping to define your curls and waves and reduce frizz. The diffuser also has long prongs, allowing you to reach deeper into your hair with better control.

Another option I love is the RevAir hairdryer (see Figure 8-9). It's the most revolutionary styling tool I've seen in years because of its design, which feels futuristic and looks like a mini vacuum cleaner, which is like no other dryer you have ever seen. It's also easy to use. As the name pays homage to, this dryer reverses the airflow. Instead of blowing, it sucks — basically, using a vacuum effect that gently stretches, straightens, and smooths all curl patterns, while at the same time removes water using very mild heat. It dries your hair 60 percent faster with heat that's 100 degrees Fahrenheit (38 degrees Celsius) cooler than traditional dryers.

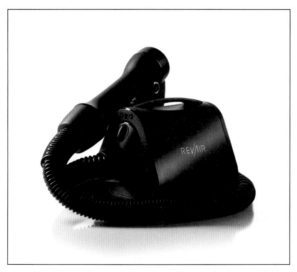

FIGURE 8-9:
The RevAir
hairdryer.

Photo courtesy of RevAir

I was mind-blown when I got a chance to use the RevAir for the first time. Honestly, I was extremely skeptical at first. I mean, the idea of sucking your hair into a tube to dry and straighten it was completely foreign to me. You don't need any attachments or blow-dry brushes when you use the RevAir, which allowed me to finish a blowout in record time. You simply place a section of wet hair in the tube and watch how quickly your hair dries and straightens with very little tension and heat (see Figures 8-10 and 8-11). It offers several levels of suctioning intensity so you can choose which level you want in order to get to your desired level of stretch. You may need to experiment.

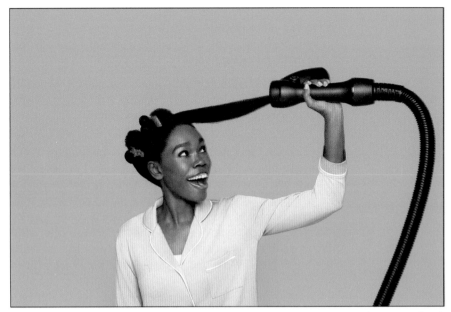

FIGURE 8-10:
The RevAir
sucks air
instead of
blowing to dry
your hair.

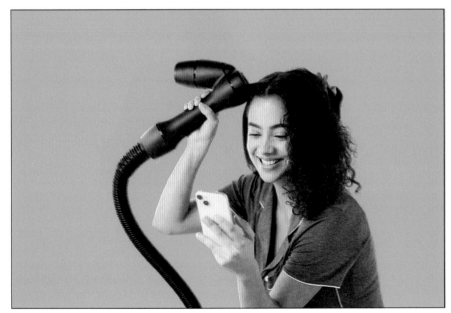

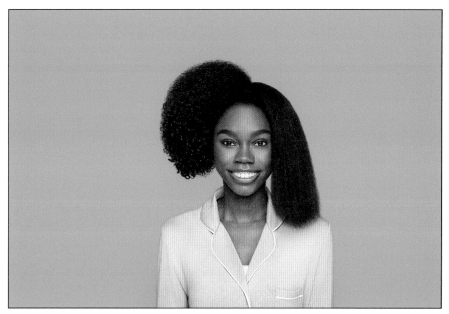

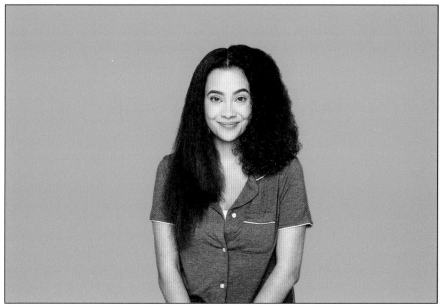

FIGURE 8-11:
Before and after using the RevAir blow dryer.

USING HOODED DRYERS

When you want to dry your hair quickly and evenly, help treatments like conditioning or protein or hot oil penetrate your hair more deeply, or set your rollers without heat damaging your hair, a hooded dryer is the way to go. A hooded dryer is a dome-shaped device that sort of looks like a helmet attached to an arm on top of a chair, and it spreads the heat out more evenly than a blow dryer, making it a gentler drying option. You usually see them in salons, but in today's world, you can buy one for your own home. At-home models come in three main types: countertop, floor, and as a bonnet-type attachment you can add onto your hair dryer. Look for a model that offers ionic technology, has a timer, has heat and speed settings you can adjust, and includes a cool setting.

The RevAir uses vacuum suctioning power and heat to dry, stretch, straighten, and smooth your hair all at the same time. Not only can you use it for your frequent or occasional blowout looks and braiding preparation, you can also use it to quickly stretch and dry twist-out styles. (RevAir LLC pays me an influencer fee to promote the RevAir hair dryer.)

TIP

Although high-quality blow dryers can be pricey, they are worth the investment. While you save up for your dream model, there's nothing wrong with selecting a more economic hair dryer that's more suitable for your pocketbook.

Hunting for a hot comb

People have been using hot combs (also known as *pressing combs*) for decades to straighten their natural and curly hair. They started as metal, manual hot combs that had wooden handles. You heated up the metal comb portion in a small thermal stove made especially for heating hot combs and Marcel curling irons of all sizes (or on a stovetop). The hot combs that you can safely use as a consumer today are electric.

Although you can use hot combs to straighten out your whole head of hair if you want, you typically use them to straighten your hairline and new growth only for particular styles, such as sleek ponytails and blowouts, and to smooth out certain areas of your lace-front wigs so that they lay more naturally.

WARNING

Don't use manual hot combs on yourself. Because of the lack of heat control, you can easily damage your hair and your skin — quickly and severely — if you don't have a lot of experience with them. Only a professional hairstylist should use these older-style manual hot tools.

If you want a hot comb for at-home use, I personally recommend the *electric pressing comb,* where electricity heats up the comb, instead of you having to use a stovetop as the heat source. When you shop for an electric hot comb, look for hot combs that have teeth placed close together because they create the tension you need to straighten properly. Also, get an electric hot comb that has variable heat control so that you can select the right amount of heat for your hair type and texture.

Here are some tips for how to use a hot comb properly:

>> Always apply a heat protectant before using hot combs.

>> Use a hot comb only if your hair is at least an inch long to avoid burning your scalp and fingers.

>> Straighten in small sections. Each section should be about 1½ to 2 inches wide.

>> While using a hot comb, start at the new growth, and use the teeth to guide you into the section of hair that you're working on. Use the base of the comb to pull the section straight.

Knowing what to look for in a curling iron or wand

Curling irons and curling wands are similar to each other, with one main difference: the design of the handle. Curling irons have the easy-to-use spring-clip handle that clamps your hair to the *barrel* (the part that heats up) while you turn. Some curling irons have the more advanced Marcel rotating handle, but still have the spring clip. Curling wands have no spring clip, so you have to wrap the sections of hair around the barrel. That's it: curling iron, clip; curling wand, no clip. Each curling tool gets the job done; you just need to figure out which tool you find more comfortable to use.

Just like flat irons (see the section "Figuring out your flat iron," earlier in this chapter), look for curling wands and irons made from ceramic, titanium, or tourmaline, and make sure they also offer variable heat control. Curling irons and wands come in several barrel sizes, and although you might add a few large curling irons to your tool collection, smaller-sized wands serve curly hair best because they mimic your curl pattern more closely (see Figure 8-12).

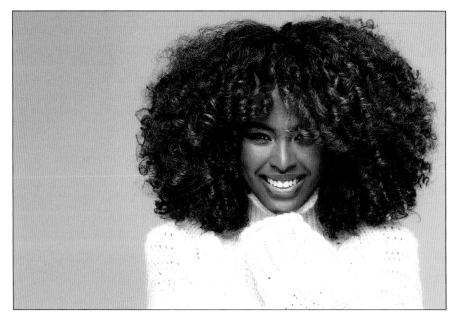

© neonshot/Adobe Stock

FIGURE 8-12:
Use a curling
iron wand
to add more
defined curls.

Small wands used on a low-heat setting help define curls and create fun textures. To do this, wrap your hair around a wand and let it sit for 5 to 7 seconds, then release. The time limit is what you need to set your curls, while the low-heat setting prevents you from causing heat damage.

REMEMBER

Although you may enjoy figuring out how to master hot tools, you must protect your hair. I can't stress enough the importance of using heat protection before you use any hot tools.

4

Creating Styles for Your Natural and Curly Hair

Create braids, twists, updos, and other styles that fully express your personality, while keeping your hair healthy and protected from harmful elements.

Use a blow dryer or flat iron to straighten your curls without heat damaging them.

Discover how to choose and install sew-ins, hair extensions, and wigs.

IN THIS CHAPTER

» **Keeping it simple with wash-and-go styling**

» **Braiding for protection and style**

» **Looking and feeling good with healthy twists and locs**

» **Caring for and wearing hair extensions and wigs**

» **Coloring and bleaching to enhance your curls**

» **Using a blow dryer to straighten or stretch your hair**

Chapter **9**

Styling Your Natural Hair

A hh, this is what I call the fun chapter. You know why? Because you have almost no limits in the creative art of natural hair styling. And because you have natural curly hair, you have so much versatility when it comes to styling options. Natural hair that hasn't been chemically treated is magical and can pretty much do anything.

In the beginning of your natural hair journey, you may feel completely lost. You not only have to figure out what products work best for you, but after years of straightening your curls, you have no idea how to style them. Whether you're newly natural or seasoned naturalista, you have no shortage of natural hairstyles to try out. Keep in mind, styling your hair requires you to develop a rhythm, so practice makes perfect, and it becomes easier the more you do it. You may go through a lot of trial and error at first, but after you get the hang of it, you'll be switching your style up all the time.

This chapter points you to a few go-to styles that you can easily create yourself in the comfort of your own home or suggest to your stylist on your next salon visit. The world is your oyster if you're open to experimenting with your beautiful curls. After you try the basic steps of a style, do it your way, and have fun with your hair.

Wearing a Wash-and-Go

When you don't want to use heat to dry your hair, you can wear a wash-and-go. A wash-and-go is almost as simple as it sounds. It's similar to a protective style because it's very low manipulation and requires low maintenance. Folks who like to keep their hair away from heat, rejoice! A wash-and-go is wearing your hair in its natural curl pattern after washing and conditioning. You can use your fingers, a detangling brush, or wide-tooth comb to detangle and apply product, but you don't use tools or anything that requires highly manipulating your hair.

To wash-and-go like a pro, follow these basic steps:

1. **Wash your hair. Blot with a towel to remove dripping excess water. But keep it wet/damp otherwise.**

   Flip back to Chapter 4 for a refresher on wash-day tips.

2. **Apply a leave-in conditioner.**

3. **Working in sections, starting at the nape of the neck, apply some styling gel, curl cream, or whatever your favorite curl-defining product is and, using your fingers, rake the product through your hair from root to ends.**

   This step helps enhance your curls or add more curl definition, especially if you have 4a to 4c hair texture. (Chapter 3 has all the details on hair texture.)

After you apply your last product, you can literally just head out the door, letting your hair air dry (see Figure 9-1).

TIP

To keep your hair wet during this process, you may need to add a little extra water, so keep a spray bottle handy.

PROTECTIVE STYLING

The more you touch, style, and manipulate your hair, the more wear and tear you put on it. To help keep your hair healthy, you can put your hair in a *protective style* — a style that's low maintenance and doesn't require you to touch it much after you put it in. The styles I cover in the sections "Braiding Your Hair" and "Twisting Your Hair," in this chapter, are inherently protective. The section "Wearing Extensions and Wigs" in this chapter also gives you extra insight about how to use them properly to protect your curls.

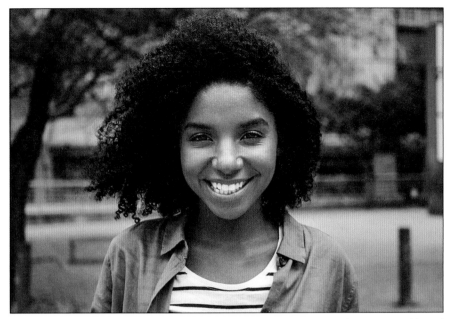

FIGURE 9-1:
Air drying your
wash-and-go
cuts down on
daily styling
time.

Braiding Your Hair

African people have been braiding their hair for centuries. Seriously, the history of hair braiding dates back to 3500 B.C. In fact, many African tribes were identified by certain braiding patterns and hairstyles. These different patterns and styles were also symbolic of someone's social status, wealth, religion and much more.

Traditionally, braiding was a bonding moment passed down through generations because of the amount of time it could take. And to this day, people still bond over hair braiding moments.

Of course, braiding has evolved over the years, particularly braids that have been sensationalized by celebrities, such as micro braids (which are super tiny braids) and fishtails (which are like cornrows, but with two strands instead of three — more on that later), but it's safe to say that hair braiding will never go out of style and will always be a go-to for naturals all around the world.

You can create braids with or without extensions. Braids (also called *plaits*) come in many patterns and sizes. You create this hairstyle by interlacing three or more sections of hair into a cylinder-like structure. When you do it properly, braiding your hair can be a good, protective styling practice and a beautiful style to wear at the same time. Braids can not only protect your hair from breakage due to constant manipulation, but — depending on how you style them — they can also look very fashionable and chic (see Figure 9-2).

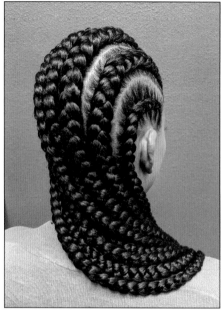

FIGURE 9-2:
Braids protect your hair from constant manipulation and can give you a sleek, polished look.

Before I get into the actual styling, here are some tools that you might need to create braids at home:

>> Blow dryer (optional)

>> Braiding hair — loose human or synthetic hair that you use to braid your hair that is not your own (optional)

>> Edge control, styling gel, or pomade

>> Wide-tooth comb

>> Rat tail comb

>> Duckbill, butterfly clips, or hair ties to secure parted sections

>> Shears for cutting/trimming braiding hair (optional)

>> Small elastic bands

>> Light oil for the scalp

Although many people find braiding a fun low-maintenance style, you absolutely must avoid any too-tight braiding styles. If you braid your hair too tightly, you can cause your scalp to itch, damage your hair strands, and in the worst cases, develop traction alopecia. *Traction alopecia* (TA) is hair loss that results from prolonged and repetitive tension on the scalp. You typically first notice TA around the front hairline while it starts to thin and recede. If you catch it early, you can reverse your TA, but if not, your hair loss can be permanent.

Follow these steps for healthy and successful braiding:

1. **Always start with freshly washed and conditioned hair.**

   Use a clarifying shampoo to remove any product buildup and residue. Then use a protein treatment followed by a hydrating conditioner to create a strong foundation for braiding (pop back to Chapter 7 if you need help choosing your products).

2. **Completely dry your hair before braiding.**

   Wet hair is more fragile. When it's wet, it expands; when it dries again, it tightens.

   You might want to straighten or stretch your hair with a blow dryer before braiding to reduce the curls, which can make it easier to braid.

TIP

3. **Use a rat tail comb for parting sections of your hair.**

   Have some hair ties and clips handy to help keep your sections separated.

4. **Apply a little edge control or your favorite pomade (something to make it tacky) to your hair shaft before braiding.**

   This type of product smooths flyaways, helps you maintain control while braiding, keeps your braids neat, and provides some added moisture to your strands.

If you start to feel any itching or notice any small bumps on your scalp (particularly around the hairline), or if your hair just feels too tight and uncomfortable after braiding, this indicates the braids are too tight. Gently comb out that braid immediately and then re-braid with less tension. The goal is taut, not too tight.

Depending or your hair type, you can wear braids for four to six weeks. When that time is up, don't repeat the same style. Changing it up to a different style helps prevent prolonged, repetitive tension on your scalp.

Box braids

Like other braiding styles, box braids have been around for centuries. Worn by several tribes from the African diaspora, they reemerged in popularity in the U.S. thanks to Janet Jackson's role as Justice in the movie *Poetic Justice* back in 1993. Fun fact: Box-braids didn't have the name recognition until Janet wore them in this movie. If you haven't seen the movie, box braids are individual braids that you section off into box-shaped divisions (see Figure 9-3).

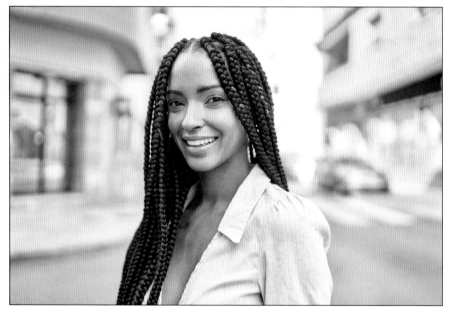

FIGURE 9-3:
Box braids.

You can do box braids yourself, especially if they are jumbo or chunky (the bigger and thicker variant of box braids), but most people get their box braids done by someone else. Depending on the speed of your stylist and the desired size and length of the braids, box braids can take from two to four hours to install. Stylists typically use loose human or synthetic hair to create these free-hanging braids, but some people ditch the extensions and braid their own hair. To do it yourself, follow these steps:

1. **Part your hair into as many square or triangular sections as you want.**
   For larger braids, do fewer sections. For smaller, do more.

2. **Divide each section into three equal parts.**

3. **Intertwine the three parts to form one single braid, twisting a silicone elastic band or hair tie around the end of each braid.**

If you go to a stylist and they use loose hair to add length and fullness, your box braids might feel a little uncomfortable and inflexible at first. To add in this loose hair, your stylist forms a knot around your hair at the base of the braid, close to the scalp, to secure the loose hair to your hair. Don't worry, they'll become more comfortable after they've had a few days to loosen up.

WARNING

If you feel a little discomfort, don't worry about it. But if you're experiencing a lot of pain, remove the braids immediately to avoid any damage. Because the knot anchors the loose hair to your natural hair, if it's installed poorly (too tight or too heavy), the box braids can cause breakage and possibly lead to TA.

Knotless braids

Knotless braids can take you (or your stylist) between four and ten hours to install, depending on the density of your hair. The time it takes to finish is substantially different from box braids because the size of knotless braids is much smaller in diameter. You start knotless braids with your natural hair and then about midway down, you feed in the loose human or synthetic hair. This approach gives your braid a seamless look, making it appear that the hair is all your own.

Because you use the feed-in technique, knotless braids apply less tension on your strands, giving you a pain-free experience and minimizing breakage.

After you install them, you can style your knotless braids right away, and you don't need to wait for them to loosen up. They're flexible immediately. Because lightweight knotless braids put less stress on your curls, you can style them however you desire.

Cornrows

I think it's safe to say that cornrows are the most popular braiding technique out there. Cornrows are perfect for summer, spring, winter, or fall. They're great for when you just don't feel like dealing with your hair in any capacity for several weeks, but still want to keep it cute (as shown in Figure 9-4). Although traditional front-to-back cornrows never go out of style, braid stylists have definitely explored their creative side and come up with some breathtaking work. It blows my mind when I think about what it takes to execute these beautiful patterns.

Cornrow hairstyles on women have a sustained popularity throughout the Somali peninsula, West Africa, and practically all of Africa as a whole. Ancient art depicting men wearing cornrow hairstyles have been traced as far back as the fifth century B.C. We see it on warriors, kings, queens, and heroes. In the U.S., cornrows came back into style during the 1960s and 1970s, and they remain popular among women, men, and children today.

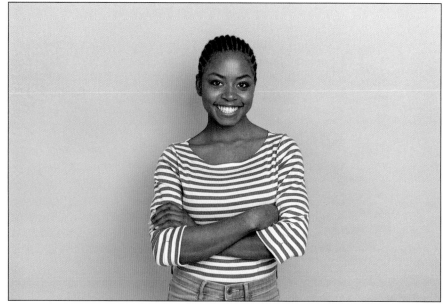

FIGURE 9-4:
Cornrows are beautiful on their own or as a foundation for crochet styles.

To give yourself cornrows, braid your hair into various patterns, from straight rows to zig-zags, close to the scalp. These braids typically mimic a cornfield — hence the name *cornrows.* You can make them any size you want. Depending on your or your stylist's skill level and the complexity of your style, cornrows can take you anywhere from 20 minutes for a simple (two to six row) style, up to four hours for a more detailed style (see Figure 9-5).

Although you can create cornrows with added human or synthetic hair, I introduce you to doing cornrows by showing you how to create a simple three-braid style that uses only your own hair. Follow these steps to put your hair in simple cornrows:

1. **Wash and detangle your hair.**

   Go back to Chapter 4 if you need a refresher on the proper wash techniques.

2. **Part your hair into three rows from front to back.**

   Make sure the middle section is evenly centered between the other two rows.

3. **Use small clips to keep the sections separated.**

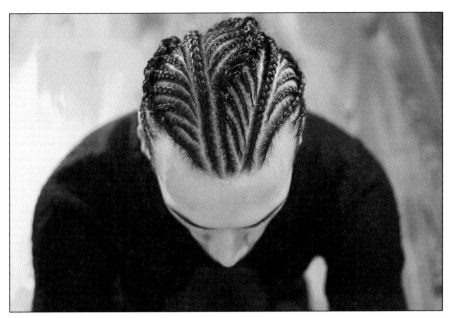

FIGURE 9-5:
Cornrows in
an intricate
design.

© gorgeoussab/Shuttterstock.com

4. **Starting near your temple on one side of your head, use your fingers to separate about an inch of hair into three evenly divided sections.**

Step 5 is optional.

5. **Apply some edge control throughout the hair if you want to tame flyaways.**

6. **Take the hair on either the left or right section and bring it over the top of the middle section.**

7. **Take the section of hair on the opposite side from the section you used in Step 6 and bring that section over the middle.**

8. **Repeat Steps 6 and 7, incorporating hair underneath the sections as you go.**

Take a little hair from under the section that you braid and add that hair to the braid to continue the cornrow and all the hair is in.

9. **After you reach the point where you no longer have hair from your scalp to add into the braid, repeat Steps 6 and 7 until you're done with that section, then secure the braid by twisting a silicone elastic band or hair tie around the end.**

10. **Repeat Steps 4 through 9 on the remaining sections created in Step 2.**

TIP

To give yourself a French braid, you can use the cornrow technique. The only difference is that you cross-section the hair under, while cornrows cross over.

Crochet technique

If you have the hang of cornrowing, you can try your hand at the crochet technique (also known as *latch hook braiding*). It's a very popular way to add extensions to your hair and is an excellent option for when you're transitioning because it's a great low-manipulation technique that allows you to grow without interruption. The crochet technique is different from sew-ins because instead of using extensions that have wefts, you use a crochet needle or hook to secure loose hair to the braids. (There's more information about extensions later in this chapter.)

Cornrows (as previously seen in Figure 9-4) act as the foundation or the base for the selected crochet style but aren't necessarily a part of the finished look of the style. Crochet styles are a great option when you're ready to protect your hair because, with a crochet style, you use little to no heat and no excessive tension.

To use the crochet technique, you first cornrow your hair, and then you use a crochet hook (yes, that kind of crochet hook as shown in Figure 9-6) to attach a hair extension to your hair. Although it takes a little practice, the technique itself isn't too difficult. To see examples of the process, search YouTube for "crochet braid technique."

FIGURE 9-6:
Use a crochet hook to loop extensions onto your cornrows.

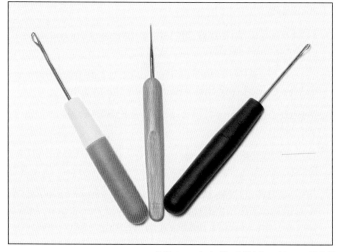

© Photography by Wardell Malloy with crowdMGMT

Goddess braids

Goddess braids are basically thicker cornrows. Like cornrows, you braid them close to your scalp, but they raise up higher because they're bigger in size. You can style them in various chic and fashionable ways for every occasion. Because of the size and the height, you pretty much always need to add loose human or synthetic hair to achieve this look.

You can also opt for goddess box braids. Goddess box braids are a softer version of traditional box braids (because they have curly tendrils that hang from the ends of the braid. The curls make the style feel effortless and carefree. You can create goddess box braids individually or by using the crochet technique.

Twisting Your Hair

Twist sets are by far the most popular go-to style for naturals across the board. You can create them easily, and you can wear them as-is or separate them into beautiful defined curls (known as a *twist out*). Twists are sort of like braids, but more simplified. Whereas you create braids with three small sections of hair, you create a twist by wrapping two small sections of hair around each other in the same direction. Normally, you create twists on damp hair while using a setting product (as shown in Figure 9-7). After you twist, you then air dry those twists or put them under a hood dryer.

Twist sets are very healthy for your hair because they don't apply any stress to your strands. You can often wear twist sets for as long as two weeks. You use the same tools as braiding to twist, so check out the supply list back in the section "Braiding Your Hair, earlier in this chapter."

Two-strand twists

With two-strand twists, you take two sections of hair and wrap them around each other in the same direction, from the roots all the way to the ends. You can do as many as you want, depending on whether you want loose or tight curls (more will yield tighter, less will yield looser). You can leave your twists as-is when you finish twisting, or you can separate them as a twist out after your hair dries. Two-strand twists work for all hair types, but they provide the most benefit in types 4a to 4c because they aid in curl definition and elongation, and 4a to 4c hair experiences a lot of shrinkage compared to the other types (see Figure 9-8).

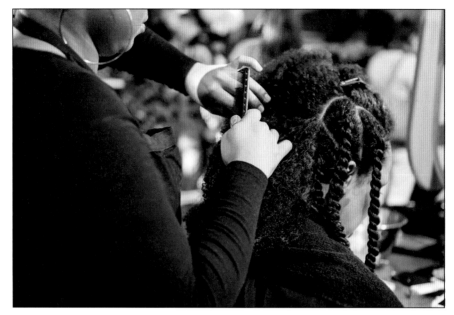

FIGURE 9-7:
A stylist can
show you how
to perfect your
twists at home.

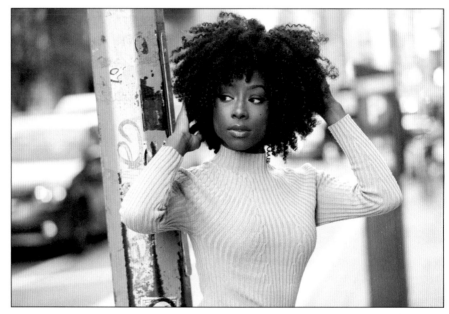

FIGURE 9-8:
Naturalistas
who have 4a
to 4c hair
can rock a
two-strand
twist like
nobody else.

Senegalese twists

Senegalese twists started in Senegal, West Africa (hence the name). These twists are great for promoting natural hair growth when you're choosing to wear a protective, low-manipulation hairstyle. *Senegalese twists* typically have a smooth, glossy finish and are very durable. (They can last for up to three months if you take care of them properly.)

You can create Senegalese twists by wrapping braiding hair around the roots of sectioned hair, and then twisting from the roots to the ends, using the two-strand twist technique as described in the preceding section.

TIP

Choose a braiding hair made from Kanekalon or Toyokalon fiber for this twist because these synthetic hairs give a smooth, glossy finish to your twists and prevent the twists from unraveling prematurely. Depending on the length of your hair, you can create these twists with your natural hair. But if you want ultimate longevity, add synthetic braiding hair.

You can install Senegalese twists in two different ways: the traditional two-strand twist technique (see Figure 9-9) and the flat-braided crochet technique. No matter which technique you choose, below are items you need for installation in addition to the tools listed in the section "Braiding Your Hair":

» Five to seven packs of synthetic braiding hair

» Latch hook crochet needle, if necessary

» Boiling water or a lighter to seal the braid ends

Traditional Senegalese twists generally take up to eight hours to install and half that time to uninstall, whereas you can install crochet Senegalese twists in four hours and uninstall them in under two hours.

Flat twists

You can create a flat twist by following the steps for cornrows, but you use two sections of hair instead of three. You can leave your hair in rows of flat twist, or separate and fluff your dry hair for a twist out. Depending on how much definition you want in your twist out, you can go with six to ten rows. More rows means smaller twists, which gives you the most curl definition. Fewer rows give you less curl definition.

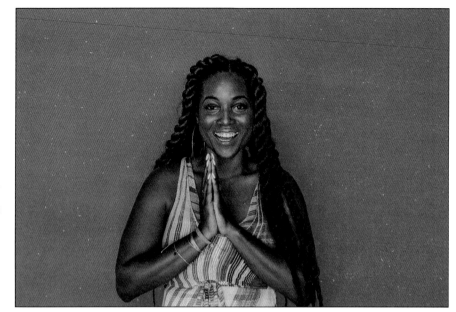

FIGURE 9-9:
There are
two different
ways to install
Senegalese
twists:
Traditional
two-strand and
flat-braided
crochet.

© Erin Brant/Stocksy/Adobe Stock

Rocking Your Locs

Locs (also called dreads, locks, and dreadlocks) is a hairstyle made up of mat-ted hair that falls into rope-like strands. Basically, locs are separate masses of interlocked kinks and knots that grow into a coil that resembles yarn. You can form these strands organically if you avoid combing and brushing your hair. Over time, your hair separates, tangles, interlocks, and meshes together to form these single rope-like strands.

Like most styling techniques, the process of starting locs has evolved over the years, and you can achieve a locked hairstyle in several ways:

>> **No manipulation/freeform:** The easiest locking technique. Just let your hair do its own thing. Simply stop combing your hair, allowing it to tangle and mesh, so that the locs form on their own. You don't need to retwist or interlock your new growth. Also, you can start these locs with practically any length of hair.

>> **Comb-twists:** The most popular technique for starting locs. Apply gel or styling cream to your hair, and then use a small-tooth comb to create cylinder-like coils by inserting the comb at the root of a section of hair and twisting the comb in a circular motion while moving down the length of the hair. You need hair that's at least 2 inches long to start comb-twists because you won't have enough hair to work with otherwise.

THE HISTORY OF LOCS

Many people wear locs as a trend or a fashion statement, not knowing the deep, rich culture and religious history they hold. Folks have worn locs since the beginning of civilization to show social power, indestructible spiritual connection, and even healing. You can trace locs back to many different cultures in history. According to scholars, kings in Africa wore locs to represent authoritative positions after winning battles, and other kings believed that locs harness energy and protected their crown chakra. (The crown chakra is in the head. It's the most spiritual of all seven chakras, and is the source of our wisdom, consciousness, and connection to higher power.) After emancipation, African Jamaicans wore locs to consciously oppose their former oppressors. Some cultures formed locs after taking vows for religious reasons to not touch their hair over a period of time. Each culture brought forth different reasons for wearing locs, and people wear them in practically every region across the world today (see accompanying photo).

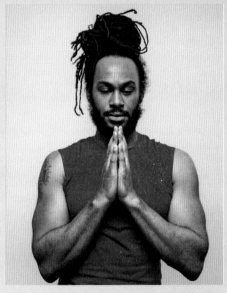

© Cavan Images/Adobe Stock

>> **Interlocking:** Essentially a crochet technique. You use a crochet hook to repeatedly pull your hair through itself near the scalp to create a base for your locs to grow and form. You can interlock in three ways: two-point, three-point, and four-point. Each rotation makes you pull your hair through the roots, using different patterns to lock your hair. You can also use this technique to create sisterlocks, which are very tiny locs. Tiny locs give you more styling

versatility than larger locs because they are closer in size to a regular hair strand. Aim to re-interlock your hair every eight weeks or so to incorporate your new hair growth.

>> **Palm rolling:** You can use this technique to help you maintain your locs as your hair grows to keep them tight and polished. Apply some locking gel to the new hair growth at the base or root of your loc. Rub your fingers back and forth to incorporate the gel and get the new hair moving. Then, flatten both of your hands like prayer hands, putting your loc in between and lightly holding. Then, roll or rub your hands back and forth so your loc rolls back and forth also. Do that until all new hair is fully incorporated, then clip the loc at the bottom until it is dry. Repeat for all your locs.

>> **Braids:** The braiding loc technique is super easy. Simply part your hair into your desired loc size, and then three-strand braid each section. Over time, the braids swell and mesh into locs when you leave them alone.

>> **Two-strand twist:** Very similar to the braiding technique, but you use two strands to twist from roots to ends.

>> **Backcombing:** Best for people who have looser curl patterns. Use a rat tail comb to tease sections of hair, then roll each section of your hair between your palms to secure each loc. To start locs this way, you need a hair length of at least 5 to 6 inches so you have enough to work with.

>> **Faux locs:** This technique uses loc extensions to avoid going through the growing phase. These extensions come in many colors, widths, and lengths, and you can attach them by using a latch hook crochet needle.

TIP

You can get more info about how to do any of these loc-starting techniques by searching for the technique of your choice online and watching tutorial videos.

Wearing Extensions and Wigs

Ah, yes — the opulent world of hair extensions. I'll be real; almost everyone wants voluminous, thick, gorgeous hair that makes them feel like they just stepped right out of a magazine. But remember, everyone has different hair textures and types, and you may not be able to easily get the look you want.

Also, many people don't want to have a stylist cut their hair really short because they simply don't have the patience for the transitioning stage. If that's you, adding hair can protect your shorter natural hair while it grows out.

From sew-ins and clip-ins to wigs, you can choose from so many options that can help add length and volume while you grow out your natural hair. Although everyone can try these options, not all of the options work for natural and curly hair. In the following sections, I share my go-to protective styles that use added hair. When you know how to do and use them properly, these styles can give your hair a break from constant manipulation, allowing it to grow with less stress on your strands.

Clip-in extensions

If you're looking to achieve length, volume, and body in just a matter of minutes, clip-in extensions can give you just what you're looking for. Clip-ins are a temporary way of attaching *wefts* (tracks of human or synthetic hair sewn onto horizontal strips of fabric, as shown in Figure 9-10) to your hair by using multiple small, pressure-point wig clips.

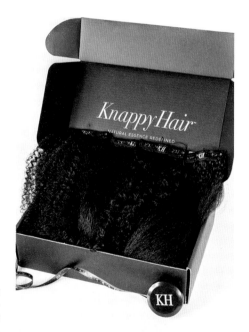

FIGURE 9-10:
Texture-
MatchKit by
KnappyHair.

Courtesy of KnappyHair Extensions

A set of clip-in extensions should include anywhere from three to ten wefts in different sizes that you can place in several areas of your head. These different sizes help you select the perfect weft to place at your nape area, high occipital bone area, sides, crown and near the hairline. You can install clip-ins very easily and remove them daily.

WARNING

Although some people decide to keep the clips in overnight, I don't recommend sleeping on them because the metal clips can cause friction on your strands while you toss and turn throughout the night. This friction can cause damage to your strands, resulting in breakage.

You can install clip-ins when your hair is in its curly state or after you blow it out straight. Follow these steps to achieve a perfect clip-in install that you can easily do in less than 30 minutes:

1. **Find clip-ins that have hair that best matches your natural hair texture.**

TIP

   Finding a good match makes the installation look more natural. Plus, the clip-ins will be versatile because you can wear them curly or straight. If you need help figuring out how many or what type of clip-ins you need, consult a salesperson — they know what they're talking about. To be clear, I feel like you can absolutely shop online for clip-ins because there is so much variety available. You can go to a website and find your perfect texture and amount. But if you feel more comfortable going to a store, by all means, do that.

2. **Use a rat tail comb to part your hair where you would like to attach (or lay) your clip-ins.**

3. **Using duckbill clips, butterfly clips, or hair ties, hold each section separately after parting in Step 2.**

   Separating each section of your hair allows you to have complete control over where you attach your wefts.

4. **Starting at the back of your head near the nape of your neck, *backcomb* (tease) your hair just a little at the roots near the parting.**

5. **Spray the teased roots with a little flexible holding spray.**

   Steps 4 and 5 give the clips a stronger foundation to latch onto in your hair, making the clips very secure.

6. **Place clip-ins about a half of an inch to an inch behind the hairline for the most natural and seamless results.**

   Make sure all the clips on the weft are open before you place them where you want to attach them.

7. **After you add enough wefts to achieve the right length and fullness, style as desired (see Figure 9-11).**

TIP

To get longevity out of your clip-in extensions, treat them with care. Remove the clips from your hair, then shampoo, condition, and gently detangle them. Lay the extensions on a flat surface to dry. You can use a blow dryer to dry your clip-ins if you're in a hurry.

I recommend washing and conditioning them about once a month. You can do it more often if you wear your clip-ins a lot or regularly apply a lot of product. Store your hair extensions in a silk or satin bag when not in use. If you properly care for your clip-ins, they can last for between six months and up to a year or more.

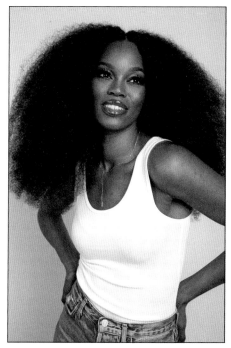

FIGURE 9-11:
Installed clip-ins from KnappyHair Extensions.

Photography by Wardell Malloy with crowdMGMT

Sew-in extensions

Throughout the years, a lot of people have turned to sew-ins for a protective style. You can use sew-ins to transition from relaxed to natural, add length and fullness, or try a completely different hair style without cutting your own hair. If you want a sew-in, I recommend that you visit a professional hairstylist for a consultation — because it's definitely a big decision to make.

When clients come to me wanting a sew-in to protect their hair, I make sure to have a thorough consultation with them. During this consultation, I examine their hair and scalp, go over pricing, and — most importantly — let them know what to expect when it comes to how long they can keep the style in.

Your stylist can install sew-in extensions (also called *weaves*) by braiding your natural hair into small (but not too small) cornrows in a particular pattern. Your stylist uses nylon thread on a needle to sew down tracks of wefted hair onto the braids. Your stylist can leave out your hairline, or center or side part to make it look more natural. Or you can get a full sew-in, which is when the base of your hair is fully braided and none of it is left out to blend with the extensions.

WARNING

Even though sew-in extensions are expensive and can take between four to six hours to install, don't wear them beyond four weeks. Yes, I said what I said — only four weeks. I know, after four weeks, it still looks good, and you want to keep it in long as possible. But while your hair grows, the weight of the extensions can start to pull on your hair strands, potentially causing breakage or traction alopecia — particularly around your hairline.

The biggest mistake I see with sew-in extensions involves making the braids too small and way too tight. Some people think that the tighter and smaller the braid, the longer it lasts. The fact is, your hair grows at the speed it grows, no matter how tight you make your braids. Too tight braids cause breakage and, in some situations, traction alopecia, which can lead to permanent hair loss. No one wants that!

If you decide to get sew-in extensions or any other protective style that requires braiding and adding extensions to your hair, have a reputable stylist, who's just as invested in the health of your hair as you are, install it. During the service, let them know if you're experiencing any pain or excessive tension from the braids. You also want to ask your stylist questions about upkeep throughout the four weeks. The more knowledge you have, the better your results. And finally, it can cost quite a coin to properly achieve the best benefits of a protective style like sew-ins, so map out your budget accordingly.

Wigs

Wigs are by far the most sought-after accessory. But sis, just because everybody and their mama is rocking a wig doesn't mean you should just pop into your local beauty supply store and slop any ol' wig on your head. You can't rush decisions like this. By taking the time to choose wigs that look natural, you can give yourself the perfect fashion statement or temporary hairstyle option.

You have two types of wigs to choose from: human hair wigs and synthetic hair wigs. Of course, the most natural-looking wigs are made with human hair because that hair lays, falls, and swings the same way the hair coming out of your head does. But if you don't want a natural-looking wig, that's your business, and I'll move on.

MY FAVORITE EXTENSIONS AND WIGS

Throughout my career, I have done thousands of sew-ins. As a stylist, I can't think of anything better than completing an install that looks natural, seamless, and literally like it's growing from your scalp. I love seeing my clients leave my chair with confidence, knowing that they won't be *clocked* when they leave the salon. Outside of laying a flat foundation (which I tell you how to do in the section "Wig installation, maintenance, and storage" later in this chapter), the hair that I choose is the most important part of the process. And using the best hair gives me flawless results. For my best hair offering, I always go with Knappy Hair Extensions.

I met Keandra Janelle (KJ), owner of Knappy Hair Extensions, during my years at the White House, and I've been obsessed with her hair ever since. KJ started her company in 2011 after she realized that she just couldn't find hair extensions that blended perfectly with textured hair if she didn't want to apply excessive heat to the hair.

KJ saw a problem that needed a solution. People of color were being forced to choose hair that didn't match their own. She noticed that typically "Brazilian," "Peruvian," and "Malaysian" descriptions didn't meet the needs of people who describe their locks as "coarse," "kinky," and "coily."

KJ researched, studied, surveyed, and traveled across the world to try to solve that problem, creating high-quality hair extensions that can blend seamlessly with kinky, coily hair. She manufactures premium hair extensions that blend beautifully with hair types 2c through 4c so that her clients don't have to waste any more time and money on hair that doesn't match their texture.

What I love most about Knappy Hair Extensions is that KJ set a new standard in the beauty industry and created a solution for a community that has been overwhelmingly underserved. Now, her brand is trusted among people who have been looking for high-quality beauty brands that understand their hair.

Knappy Hair Extensions offers an array of beautiful options to help you find the right match for your textured hair (see the accompanying photo). So, if you want to try

(continued)

(continued)

clip-ins, sew-ins, and all kinds of wigs in your kinky, coily hair, visit www.krshairgroup.com and discover hair that lets you feel like you.

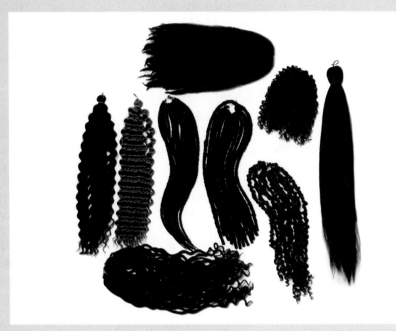

Photography by Wardell Malloy with crowdMGMT

Wigs come in different forms:

>> **Full wigs:** Cover your entire head. You tuck all of your natural hair into them, and you don't have to blend any of your hair with the wig.

>> **Half wigs:** Cover only part of your head. Half wigs allow you to frame your face with your natural hair. These wigs blend seamlessly with your natural hair while adding fullness and length to the crown and the back.

>> **Fall wigs:** Right in between full wigs and half wigs, these wigs "fall" just behind the hairline and blend with your natural hair.

TIP

You can find readymade wigs in most beauty supply stores. These wigs are one-size-fits-all, and you can adjust them to fit your head with the adjustable elastic bands inside. They come in all hair types, textures, and lengths. And they also come in a range of prices, based on the features of the wig. A really good, basic synthetic wig can cost between $50 and $150, and human hair wigs can range between $75 and $500.

Although you can find a wide selection of gorgeous readymade wigs, to get the most natural-looking wig, invest in a custom-made piece. Custom wigs are hand-made, typically by a hairstylist or wig maker who takes several measurements of your head form and builds a wig that's tailored to your head and face shape. Then they sew or hand-tie (or both) the hair of your choice to a lightweight wig cap or laced-based foundation that fits your head perfectly. Because of the detailed labor required to create them, and depending on the materials used, custom-made wigs can cost anywhere from $1,300 to as high as $20,000 or more.

A little about lace front wigs

Since the release of Beyoncé's debut album, *Dangerously In Love,* in 2003, lace front wigs have taken center stage. Yes, over the past 20 years or so, lace front wigs have evolved tremendously and have practically taken the spot of the coveted relaxer in the beauty industry. Wig makers craft lace front wigs to mimic your natural hairline. Hair strands are individually hand tied into a thin, almost invis-ible, lace material at the hairline and frontal crown area. Originally created for theater, film, and television to help build a character, the lace around the hairline of the wig imparts realism to the hairstyle while looking natural because it blends with your skin tone and gives the illusion that the hair is growing from the scalp. Today, lace front wigs are worn by almost everyone and, when installed properly, can look like your natural hair. You can style them the same way you'd style your natural hair — with various cuts, part sections, and even ponytails or braids.

Although wigs provide an excellent option for people experiencing excessive thinning and hair loss, naturals can also benefit from wigs because wigs protect hair from daily styling manipulation. However, if you wear your wig too much, it can cause friction and erode your hairline, which can lead to TA.

Wig caps

If you want to prevent thinning or breakage, wear your wigs in moderation and always place a wig cap on your head before placing the wig.

Wig caps are thin, soft caps that stretch and fit over your head. Your hair can tuck up and under the cap, which creates a smooth foundation by helping keep hair in place underneath the wig. The wig cap also acts as a layer of protection for your natural hair by reducing friction between the wig and your hair, while creating friction for the wig to help it grip the cap and stay in place.

Even if you have total hair loss, use a wig cap to prevent your wig from slipping off and as a barrier to protect your sensitive scalp from potential irritation from the wig's interior material sitting directly on your head. Ultimately, wearing a wig cap gives you a more comfortable wig-wearing experience.

Most wig caps come as one-size-fits-all because they're made of elastic material that can stretch to fit nearly any head, but you might find an elastic wig cap too tight after wearing one for a long period of time. If you find an elastic wig cap uncomfortable, just go without one.

Wig installation, maintenance, and storage

You don't have to put in a lot of effort to install and wear full, half, and fall wigs.

FOUNDATION

First, create a good foundation for your wig to attach to and sit on. Which technique works best for attaching your wig depends on your hair length. If you have short hair, brush it down as flat as possible (use styling gel, if needed), then cover it with a wig cap. If you have longer hair, pull your hair back in a smooth, low ponytail or small-to-medium cornrows that go from the front to the back of your head. Then cover your hair with a wig cap. In the end, you want a foundation that's as flat and smooth as possible. After you have your foundation ready, you can attach your wig.

INSTALLATION

Wigs have small combs or clips around the inside perimeter that grip to your hair or wig cap, securing the wig in place. You just have to place your wig how you want it, then push the combs or clips into your wig cap or hair.

Lace front wigs are a little more complicated to install because you need double-sided tape or wig glue (and a little skill) to attach them correctly. The double-sided tape or wig glue attaches the lace to your head nearly invisibly.

Of course, a professional can give you the best results for lace front wig services, but if you want to try installing one yourself, follow these steps:

1. **Shampoo, condition, and dry your hair.**

    Refer to Chapter 7 to select the best products to keep your covered hair healthy.

2. **Create your foundation as described in the previous section called "Foundation."**

    Don't put your wig cap on yet.

3. **Wipe alcohol pads on your skin in front of your hairline where you want to place the lace front.**

    If your skin doesn't have any oils or products on it before you apply the wig glue, you get better adhesion.

4. **Smooth your hairline back by using styling gel or pomade.**

5. **Place a wig cap over your head.**

    The section "Wig caps," earlier in this chapter, discusses the details about getting the right wig cap.

6. **Spray a strong-hold hairspray on top of the wig cap right at the hairline to secure the cap in place. The spray will soak through to your scalp and will hold the cap in place.**

7. **Trim off the excess fabric from the forehead using sharp shears. Go slowly and work your way around.**

8. **Place the wig on your head, then gently adjust it to where you want the wig to sit.**

    The lace should sit right in front of your natural hairline.

9. **After you get the wig where it feels comfortable for you, cut the excess lace from around the ear and hairline with sharp shears. Go slowly and work your way around.**

10. **Use duckbill clips to hold the front of your wig away from your forehead and temple area. Fold your wig back a little and clip it straight on and back to hold it out of your face.**

11. **Place the wig glue right at the edge of the wig cap.**

    Don't put the wig glue directly on your natural hairline because the glue can rip out your edges when you remove the wig.

12. **Blow dry the glue on a cool setting.**

    Dry the glue until it's a little tacky but not stringy.

13. **After the wig glue dries, remove the duckbill clips and gently pull the wig.**

14. **Place the lace on top of the glue, making sure it's exactly where you want it, then firmly press the lace into the glue.**

15. **Use alcohol wipes to remove any extra glue on your forehead.**

    Avoid wiping the lace because it would loosen or remove the glue under the lace.

16. **Tie a narrow satin or silk scarf around your hairline and allow the glue to dry completely.**

    The lace will "melt" into your skin seamlessly, so you can't tell it's not your natural hairline.

17. **Style your lace front wig as desired.**

Installing lace front wigs provides a pretty decent challenge, so don't feel discouraged if it doesn't go well on your first try. Just keep practicing. Here are some of my favorite tips to help you successfully install:

>> When using a wig cap, use a skin-tone concealer in any parted areas before you place the wig to help blend the lace to match your skin.

>> For a more secure installation, use a needle with nylon thread to sew over the top of the wig and from ear to ear around the back of the wig.

>> Always use an adhesive remover to take off the wig glue and follow the manufacturer's instructions.

>> Use tweezers to pluck hair from the wig along the hairline and partings to mimic a more natural-looking appearance. You can do this before or after you place the wig.

>> Try to place the lace as close to your hairline as possible without overlapping. Don't make your forehead a "two-head" because you place your lace too far down.

NON-GLUE WIG OPTIONS

Not all lace front wigs require wig glue. As I mention in the section "Installation," earlier in this chapter, you can use lace front wig tape, which is double-sided tape, instead of wig glue to secure your wigs. Tape has less of a chance of damaging your hairline. Just follow the same steps as gluing. First, wipe your head with alcohol to remove any oil or residue so the tape sticks to your skin well. Then, lay the tape along the hairline of the wig and place the wig where desired.

You can also use glueless wigs. These full lace wigs don't require any type of adhesive to attach. You secure the wig by using bands, combs, or clips, and the lace lays flat on your forehead without the need for glue or tape. Glueless wigs let you avoid putting adhesives anywhere near your hairline, but get a custom-made wig so that the wig's lace hairline can lay perfectly.

The process for maintaining and storing wigs is pretty easy and straightforward:

>> **Wigs:** After you wear your wig for a while, it may start to look limp and doesn't move like it did when it was fresh. It's probably time to shampoo. Simply remove the wig and, using the same products you use on wash day (see Chapter 7), shampoo and condition (and detangle, if needed). Then rinse and towel dry your wig thoroughly. Place your wig on a Styrofoam or a cork wig head to dry. The wig head helps keep the wig's shape and allows the hair to dry how it naturally falls.

> » **Lace front wigs:** Use adhesive remover to safely remove the wig from your head, then follow the same steps in the preceding bullet. You may need to keep the adhesive remover handy while you shampoo the wig to help lift off any glue still on the lace. Use wig pins to hold the wigs in place on the wig head.

TIP

Use a blow dryer to dry your wig if you're planning on wearing it immediately.

Coloring and Bleaching Natural and Curly Hair

In the past, coloring and bleaching textured hair wasn't as popular as it is today. For years, people found maintaining colored (particularly bleached) relaxed or natural hair nearly impossible. Some people could achieve great results with reds, warm shades of blonde (see Figure 9-12), and (of course) darker colors such as black and browns for gray coverage. But most people didn't dare try vivid colors, which required you to bleach your hair first before depositing the tone, which could have led to major or permanent damage.

Thank the hair gods — times have changed. The popularity of styling products for natural and curly hair means you can find many options designed for the textured hair community so that you can experiment with an array of permanent colors and bleaching. From jet black to icy platinum blondes, brands such as Olaplex have changed the color game by implementing innovative technology in their products that helps protect and nourish the hair during the coloring process. More brands than ever recognize this need and continue to develop permanent hair care products that are safe for textured hair. Now, people who have natural and curly hair who want to experiment with unique hues don't have to settle for the limited selection of semi or demi colors, which are colors that simply sit on top of the hair strand and give it the illusion of the hair having another color.

WARNING

Although you can apply semi and demi colors safely and easily at home, always leave permanent hair coloring and bleaching in the hands of the professionals. Permanent hair coloring is a process that uses ammonia to permanently change the color of your hair. During this process, your natural pigment is removed and replaced by artificial pigment. As you can imagine, if you don't do it properly, you can cause a lot of damage. And truthfully, you have no way of knowing whether your hair can handle a coloring process, but a professional can tell. So again, *please leave permanent hair coloring and bleaching in the hands of a professional!*

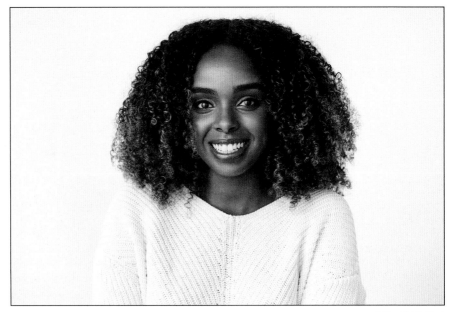

FIGURE 9-12:
If you want
safe and
effective hair
color, visit a
professional.

For more information about caring for your color-treated hair, flip back to Chapter 6.

Getting Your Hair Cut

You may want a haircut for all different reasons. You may want a new look, to try a new trend, or to get fresh, low-maintenance look as shown in Figure 9-13.

Over the years, stylists have had a huge debate about whether to cut curly hair in its natural state or after you blow it out straight. Leave that debate to professional hairstylists. For me, I do a mixture of both techniques. I like to cut and create the length and most of the shape when the hair is blown out, then define the shape after I diffuse the curls.

However your stylist prefers to cut, stick with the pros: Don't go botching up your hair by trying to cut it yourself. As hairstylists, we spend years perfecting our craft to give you a beautiful cut that shapes your face perfectly and adds to the illustration of your personal story. So, when you want to try a shorter haircut or you need your next trim, treat yourself and let a stylist do what we love to do. If you want information on trimming, refer back to Chapter 6.

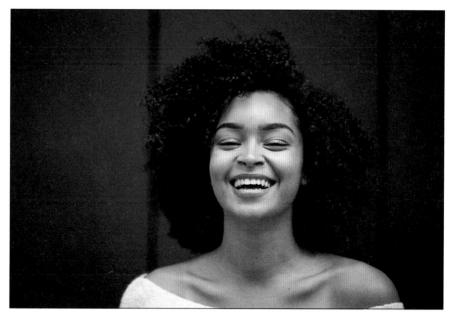

FIGURE 9-13:
A stylist can give you a cut that is low maintenance.

Blowing Out Your Hair

In my opinion, one of the best things about natural curly hair is its versatility. I love that you can go from a big, frizzy afro to bone straight, and everything in between. Blowing out your hair is probably one of the most dramatic changes you can make to your curls in under an hour. With the right techniques and tools, you can do it safely at home. Although blow drying natural hair many times gets a bad rap in the natural–hair community, if you do it properly, you can reduce tangles, stretch out stubborn kinks, and make your hair appear longer.

If you want to straighten your hair with a blow dryer, you need

» Heat protectant and/or blow-dry smoothing balm products

» Rat tail comb or wide-tooth comb to part your sections

» Duckbill or butterfly clips to hold the wet hair away from the drying hair

» Powerful blow dryer that has multiple heat settings

» Blow-dry brush like a Denman or a paddle brush or just use the comb attachment on your blow dryer

DOING BLOWOUTS WITH LESS TENSION

Most natural textures have a lot of shrinkage, and with all the bends and curls, your hair can draw up tight to your scalp. Adding an additional step to your blow drying allows you to pull the hair straight while it dries so that you can apply less tension with the blow-dry brush. This reduced tension, in turn, preserves your curls and reduces damage caused by the blow-drying process. You can use this technique with a traditional blow dryer by gently pulling the section straight with one hand while the other hand holds the blow-dryer. Move the blow dryer up and down about 2 to 3 inches away from the section until the hair is about 75 percent dry. Then, pull the hair completely straight with the blow-dry brush while you finish drying your hair with the blow dryer.

To straighten your hair at home, follow these steps:

1. **Shampoo and condition your hair.**

2. **Towel dry your hair.**

   Don't overdo it. Leave your hair pretty damp.

3. **Add a heat protectant or smoothing balm.**

   Either spray it or apply a small amount to your hands and distribute evenly by raking your fingers through your hair.

4. **Section your hair.**

   You can either separate your hair into four to six sections, drying each section one at a time, or you can start at the nape of your neck and dry small horizontal sections.

5. **Use the blow-dry brush to grip a section of your hair. Place the hairdryer nozzle on top of your hair.**

6. **Gently pull your brush and dryer straight down through your hair.**

7. **Repeat Steps 5 and 6 for each section of hair.**

   Work your way upwards, drying each section until you dry all the hair on your head.

8. **Style your straightened hair as desired (see Figure 9-14).**

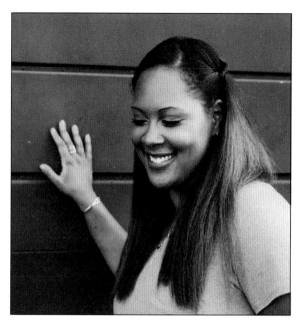

FIGURE 9-14:
Use a blow-
dryer to
straighten your
curls for even
more styling
versality.

© nappy/Pexels

HOW TO FIND A PROFESSIONAL HAIRSTYLIST

If you scroll through social media, you don't find a shortage of stylists who post amazing images of hair extension and wig work that they've done. In fact, #lacefrontal, #lacefrontwigs, and #lacefrontinstall are all popular hashtags that can point you in the right direction. Outside of recommendations from a friend, if you want to find a great stylist, social media gives you one of the best places to see someone's work. Many stylists offer a portfolio of images that showcase their craft through various social media platforms. After you do your due diligence, go ahead and slip into those DMs and book a consultation to see if you and the stylist make a good fit.

A consultation gives you not only a chance to see a stylist's work in person, but also to gauge their salon environment and professionalism, as well as ask as many questions as you want. A perfect fit can answer all your questions effortlessly. If you're not feeling the vibe, scratch them off your list and move on to the next one. For more info on finding a stylist, go back to Chapter 6.

One of the most innovative tools to add to your collection is the RevAir reverse hair dryer. Ever since RevAir hit the market in 2018, I've been continuously amazed at the results I get when I use this dryer. It's revolutionary, and you can't find anything else on the market like it. RevAir gives you the power and flexibility to stretch and blow-out your hair in a healthy way, without high heat and with minimal tension, in just a fraction of the time that traditional drying methods need. The reverse-air technology dries, stretches, and straightens hair three times faster than a traditional blow-dryer. I believe that RevAir provides a healthier drying choice than the more traditional methods, giving naturally curly, wavy, coily, and kinky hair textures mind-blowing results. The aerodynamically designed wand can easily dry any type of hair, including coarse hair, braids, locs, and extensions, leaving the hair smooth and ready to style, or prepped for a protective style. See Chapter 8 for more information.

REMEMBER

In a highly filtered world, never trust what you see on social media. Always do a consult before styling, no matter how great the photos look.

IN THIS CHAPTER

» **Creating updos and sealing your braids**

» **Styling your twists and Bantu knots**

» **Wearing your hair in an afro**

» **Making a bun**

» **Adding head wraps to your styling options**

Chapter **10**

Quick and Easy Style Ideas

I said it before, and I'll say it over and over again: The most amazing gift you get from going natural is versatility. When you have natural and curly hair, it's not about wearing only one particular style; it's about always having multiple options and the ability to switch your style up according to your mood and vibe at any given moment.

This chapter takes the braiding styles from Chapter 9 a step further by providing some options for creating additional easy-to-do styles so that you can go on with your day. You don't have any rules when it comes to trying to create a hairstyle. So whatever style you choose to rock, as long as you keep your curls healthy, you can't find a wrong way to style it.

REMEMBER

Everyone has their own unique curl pattern, so focus on simulation, not duplication. What I mean by that is, when you see a style that you want to try, go for it! Just realize that no two people are exactly the same, so that style will look slightly different on you, no matter how hard you try to make it an exact copy. Embrace how your hair expresses the same style in its own unique way.

Styling Your Braids

All over the world, women, men, and children wear braids — just as they have for thousands of years. On the playground, in the office, or at an elegant affair, braids are perfect for any occasion and can protect your hair as a low-manipulation style.

Like I talk about in Chapter 9, you have a lot of braiding options to try, but the most popular types of braids for naturals are

>> Box braids

>> Micro braids (see Figure 10-1)

>> Cornrows

>> French braids

>> Fishtail braids

>> Crochet braids

>> Knotless braids

>> Chunky/jumbo box braids

>> Goddess braids

I encourage you to go to YouTube and type your braid of interest into the search bar, and then watch as many of the videos that pop up as needed to help you create and/or style these braids.

Braided updos

Back in the day, elaborate updos were reserved for black-tie affairs, but today, people commonly wear their curls in a creative updo style even on a regular day (see Figure 10-2). Whether you *snatch* braids back into a single ponytail, pull them up in a top knot, wear them half up/half down, put them in a bun, or sweep them to the side, styling updos out of your braids gives you a polished, clean, and effortless look that can have a casual, elegant, and even vintage appeal.

Updos not only can look like a work of art, but also help you keep cool and still look your best on those hot days.

Because you have so many different easy-to-create updos for various lengths of natural hair to choose from, surf the Internet and look for styles that speak to you. Then just give them a try. Or visit a natural hairstylist who specializes in updos and can help you save some time and energy.

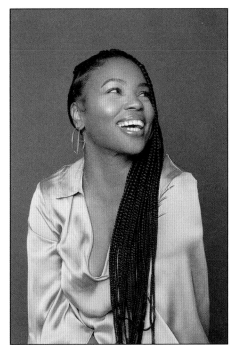

FIGURE 10-1:
Micro braids
can give the
illusion of
individual hair
strands.

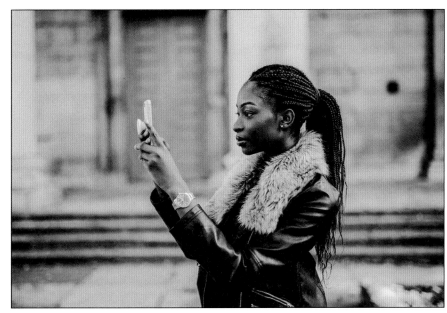

FIGURE 10-2:
Braids can be
pulled back
into a ponytail
using loose
hair ties.

The best thing about creating an updo with your braided hair is that there are no rules to when you have to do it. You can do it on freshly cleaned or days-old braids. If you want to try an updo, here are some tips before you get started:

>> **Visualize what you're trying to create.** This is where Pinterest, YouTube, Instagram, and magazines come in handy. Having an idea of where you're going helps you achieve your desired look (see Figure 10-3).

>> **Decide which texture you want for your updo.** You can leave your hair in its natural state after you shampoo, condition, and air dry it (or after separating your twists and braids), or you can use the stretching technique to gently stretch out your curls.

>> **Be prepared and organized.** Have all of your products and tools easily accessible so that you don't waste time searching for things while you have your hands in your hair. Depending on the style, you might need items such as silicone elastic bands or hair ties (for hair types 4a–4c, use satin or silk hair ties), duckbill clips, a rat tail comb, and edge control.

>> **Work in sections.** Working in sections is key for new naturals because it keeps you from feeling too overwhelmed.

The more you get to know your hair and all the fun things you can do with it, the more easily you can create unique styles. Over time, you can get comfortable enough that you don't need to work in sections.

>> **Secure your updo properly.** Of course, you have a trusted hair tie among your styling accessories, but you should also have a variety of hair pins and bobby pins on deck (see the sidebar "Hair pins versus bobby pins," in this chapter) to guarantee your 'do stays up.

>> **Enjoy yourself.** Finally, and most importantly, just have fun creating!

Crochet styles

You can find many crochet styles out there. Here are a few of the most common styles:

>> **Crochet twist outs:** Give you the look of a natural hair twist out

>> **Faux locs:** Great if you want to try locs but don't want to fully commit to them just yet (see Figure 10-4)

>> **Crochet box braids:** More simple and faster to install than traditional box braids, but you get a similar look

>> **Crochet Senegalese twists:** Give a smooth, defined look

>> **Crochet Havana twists:** The way to go if you like big and thick braids

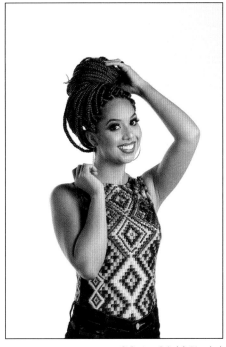

FIGURE 10-3:
Determine the placement of your braids in an updo before you add bobby pins.

I provide instructions on cornrows and the crochet technique in Chapter 9. In this chapter, I just give you a little extra insight that you can use to find the right type of hair extensions and how to use them to create different styles.

You can purchase two different types of crochet hair extensions:

» **Synthetic:** More popular than human hair because it's very affordable, easy to install and style, and comes in a variety of colors and textures. Synthetic crochet hair extensions are denser than real hair and don't slip as much, so you can keep your style longer.

» **Human:** Best for people who want to style their crochet style similar to their own hair. You can use any heat styling tool to create your look without fear of the hair melting. Plus, human hair extensions give you a great alternative if you're allergic to synthetic hair. (You might not realize you are allergic until you come into contact with it. You may experience irritation as a result.) I want to warn you, though, that using human hair for your crochet style comes with a few issues:

  • *Time:* Real hair is slippery, so it loosens and falls out faster than synthetic hair. And when you're trying to get as much use as you can from your style, that's not cool.

  • *Money:* Human hair extensions cost way more than synthetic extensions.

HAIR PINS VERSUS BOBBY PINS

Hair and bobby pins come in a few different lengths and sizes. Trust me, get them all! You can find a use for every size. Bobby pins (a) are closed at the tip and bumpy on one side, whereas hair pins (b) are like an elongated U, and both sides are bumpy. They should both have tiny balls at the ends that you insert into your hair. These tiny balls and bumpy sides help the pins to grip the hair and stay in place.

As for bobby pins, in some instances, you may wish to open the pins first. Then insert the pins, and wiggle them in, instead of simply sliding them in. This little wiggle helps the pins grip the hair better and keeps your updo feeling secured in place.

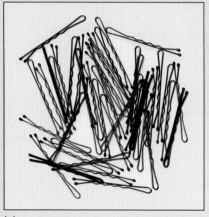

(a) *Photography by Wardell Malloy with crowdMGMT*

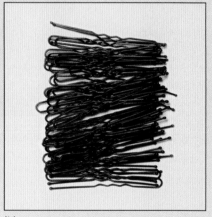

(b) *Photography by Wardell Malloy with crowdMGMT*

As you can see in Figures 10-5 through 10-7, crochet hair comes in a few different textures, including

» **Straight:** Great for people who like switching it up because you can wear it straight or restyle it with light heat. These extensions can give you that straight, sleek, blown-out look without the threat of any heat damage to your own hair. You can style it in a ponytail or a cute updo, or you can wear it down and let it fall beautifully down your back and over your shoulders.

Some synthetic straight hair can handle a little heat. Just check the package for instructions.

» **Wavy:** If your natural hair texture is on the curlier side, wavy crochet extensions are the way to go when you want to experiment with something different. With this texture, you can wake up and go without putting much effort into styling.

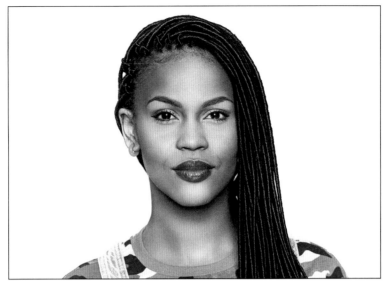

FIGURE 10-4:
Smooth
faux locs.

>> **Curly:** Perfect for when you simply want to give your own curls a break from daily manipulation and when you need a break from your daily routine. It comes in a variety of curl patterns and looks great short or long.

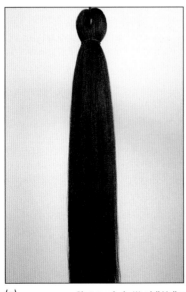

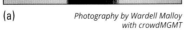

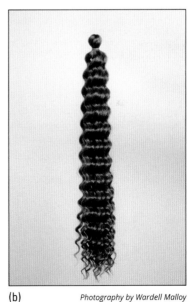

FIGURE 10-5:
Straight (a),
wavy (b).

(a) *Photography by Wardell Malloy with crowdMGMT*

(b) *Photography by Wardell Malloy with crowdMGMT*

>> **Twist:** Crochet twisted extensions come in several different twist forms; two strand twists and Senegalese twists (flip back to Chapter 9 for more on these). This texture gives you the look of a natural twist.

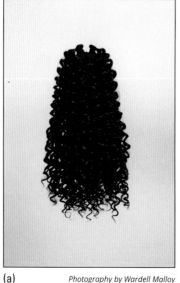 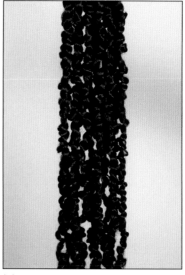

FIGURE 10-6:
Curly (a),
twists (b).

(a)   *Photography by Wardell Malloy with crowdMGMT*   (b)   *Photography by Wardell Malloy with crowdMGMT*

>> **Braids:** Come pre-braided, which gives you a great option if you want to try the box braids look but don't have or want to take the time needed to sit for hours getting them done to your own hair. Crochet box braids take half the time for installation and take down, which varies for everyone.

>> **Faux locs:** I love locs, and out of all the crochet textures, faux locs are my favorite because they require less commitment than natural locs. Natural locs truly require almost a spiritual level of commitment because they take years to grow, whereas faux locs can be installed in a few hours.

While you wear a crochet hairstyle, please show your scalp some love. Here are some tips:

>> Use a lightweight oil to keep your scalp moisturized.

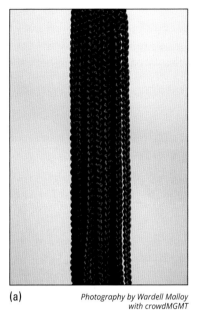
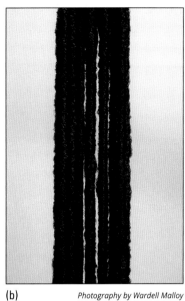

FIGURE 10-7:
Braids (a), faux
locs (b).

(a) *Photography by Wardell Malloy with crowdMGMT*

(b) *Photography by Wardell Malloy with crowdMGMT*

WARNING

>> Minimize frizz and keep your style fresh by lightly spraying a shine spray on the crochet hair when it starts to look dry or needs refreshing.

Don't spray too much or too often because too much and too often will add too much product, which weighs the hair down.

>> To get the most out of your crochet style, always sleep with a silk or satin head covering or pillowcase. Go back to Chapter 6 if you need a refresher on how to protect your hair while you sleep.

Sealing your braids

I want to share some insight about sealing the ends of your braids. You want get the most longevity out of your style so that the time you spent to create them isn't in vain.

REMEMBER

If your braids aren't sealed correctly, they unravel at the ends.

Hot water

You can use hot water to seal your synthetic hair braids. Be extremely careful and take your time because you are working with very hot water and could burn yourself if you try to rush it. You need a large jug for the water and a dry towel handy. Just follow these steps:

1. **After you finish your braids, separate them into four sections so that you can easily manage and control them.**

2. **Boil a gallon of water to a temperature of 190 degrees Fahrenheit (87 degrees Celsius), then pour the water into the large jug.**

   Put the jug on a stable surface like a table or countertop.

3. **Dip about 3 to 5 inches of one section of braids into the jug of water and hold them there for 10 to 15 seconds.**

4. **Carefully pull them out of the water and onto the dry towel.**

5. **Dab the water off with the towel.**

6. **Hold your braids in the towel for about 20 more seconds while they cool down.**

7. **Repeat Steps 3 through 6 with the remaining sections.**

TIP

Watch a stylist do this before you attempt it yourself. Search online for example videos.

A flat iron

If you use synthetic hair and don't want to use hot water, you can just as effectively seal off your ends by using a flat iron. Follow these steps:

1. **Set a flat iron to high heat not to exceed 400 degrees Fahrenheit (204 degrees Celsius).**

2. **Pull a small piece of hair away from the end of the braid where you want to seal it.**

3. **Loop those strands around the braid at the bottom four to five times.**

4. **Hold the strands away from the braid and grip firmly.**

5. **Place the corner of the flat iron over the looped area for a few seconds.**

6. **While the synthetic hair melts and seals, wiggle the loose strands away from the rest of the braid.**

7. **Remove the braid from the iron and roll the sealed area between two fingers a few times while cooling to really finish the sealing.**

When using this technique, each braid has to be sealed individually since you only have two hands to work with!

TIP

If there's any residue left behind by the hair, wait until the iron cools, unplug it, and clean it with soft towel dipped in water or rubbing alcohol.

Glue

If you don't feel comfortable using any type of heat to seal your braids, you can instead use nail glue or super glue. Just use the glue sparingly to avoid leaving a small white stain on your braid. To use glue, follow these steps:

1. **Braid almost to the end of the braid, past where your natural hair ends.**

2. **Dab a small drop of glue on the middle of the three strands.**

3. **Braid over the drop of glue to lock it in.**

TIP

Be mindful and careful not to get any glue on your hands because it's hard to get off!

Styling Options for Twists

I mean, what's not to love about twists? They work for all hair types, they're great for the times you want a protective style, they're pretty low-maintenance, and you can easily to do them yourself. Like the name suggests, twists involve wrapping different sections of your hair around themselves in a spiral or twist pattern. (I cover the how-to steps in Chapter 9). Because twist styles are so versatile, it's practically impossible to get bored with them.

In the following sections, I give you a couple of options for styling your twists.

Twist outs

The number one tip to remember when you want a perfect twist out is: The more you let it dry, the better. Always let your twists dry completely to get the best results. Depending on how long or thick your hair is and how much time you need for it to dry completely, I recommend following these steps:

1. **Use the LOC (liquid, oil, cream) method to moisturize your hair and help with curl definition. Flip back to Chapter 4 for more info.**

2. **Twist your hair in the evening.**

3. **Sit under a hooded dryer so that you can get your hair between 50 to 70 percent dry.**

4. **Cover your twist with a satin or silk bonnet or scarf, and let your hair continue to dry overnight while you sleep.**

5. **In the morning (or whenever you like), untwist your hair.**

6. **Using the balls of your fingertips, gently massage the lines of demarcation out of your hair at the parts.**

Allowing your twists to be 100 percent dry before taking them apart gives you longer-lasting curl definition.

TIP

After you master two-strand twists, try the three-strand twists. Similar to braids, you use three sections (or strands) of hair. Instead of crossing the strands in opposite directions, the three strands are twisted in the same direction. You can wear them as is or unravel the twists when they're completely dry for even more defined curls.

Flat twist out

One of the most versatile — and, in my opinion, easiest — styles is the flat twist out (more on flat twists back in Chapter 9). It offers maximum curl definition without excessive tension or breakage, and it holds up pretty well between wash days. And with flat twists, you can switch up the direction and size. You typically place flat twists away from your face, but you can also place them towards your face or up into a ponytail, mohawk, updo, and even swept to the side.

You can wear flat twists as is for a few days; when done properly, a flat twist can last up to seven to ten days. It offers a perfect option for those times when you don't want to touch your hair much throughout the week. Then you can unravel the twists to reveal beautifully defined curls so that you can rock a twist out for a few more days.

Here are a few tips to help keep your twist out or flat twist out looking fresh between wash days:

>> **Start your twist with wet hair.** When you do your initial twist while your hair is damp, your twist sets better and lasts longer. Be sure to apply detangler thoroughly to your hair before you start your twist.

>> **Use the liquid, oil, and cream (LOC) method to moisturize before you twist.** Ensure that your hair stays hydrated and keeps its natural shine between wash days. For more on the LOC method, flip to Chapter 4.

>> **Wait until your hair is completely dry before you take the twists apart.** When you unravel twists while they're still damp, your hair has more frizz and less curl definition.

>> **Use a light oil at night before going to bed.** If you feel like your curls look a little parched after a few days, gently apply your favorite light oil before covering it up for bed. Need help choosing an oil? Visit Chapter 7.

>> **Use the chunky twist method (twisting only four or five sections) or the pineapple method to help maintain your curls overnight.** Depending on the length and/or density of your hair, either method can help keep the twist shape by preventing the smooshing effect of resting your head on your hair while you sleep. So either method can help you keep curl definition. Visit Chapter 5 for more on the pineapple method.

>> **Protect your curls while you sleep.** Satin or silk head coverings and pillowcases are your best friends while you're wearing twists. They minimize frizz, and your curls will look so happy in the morning.

>> **Avoid excessive touching.** Give your hair a little break. Touching your hair over and over kind of defeats the purpose of a low-manipulation style.

Rocking Bantu Knots

Bantu knots are a stylish way to elevate your look — and they are easier to do than you might think. The basic idea involves separating your hair into several small sections, and then twisting each section up and around itself to make a little bun or knot. Follow these steps to use this protective style:

1. **Shampoo, detangle, and condition your hair.**

   You can get the scoop on wash day in Chapter 4.

2. **Part your hair into multiple sections.**

   The number of sections is totally up to you. You can use a rat tail comb and duckbill clips to help you with this step (go back to Chapter 8 if you want the details on these tools).

3. **Take a small segment of one section of hair and use one hand to hold the base of it.**

4. **Use your other hand to wind your hair around itself into a knot.**

   You can also use a two-strand twist if you prefer, and then wind the twist. Aim for it to be firm — not too loose, not super tight.

   If you need extra help getting your knot to stay together or look smooth, use a gel or pomade.

5. **Tuck the end of your hair into the knot with your finger or the end of the rat tail comb.**

6. **Secure the knot with a bobby pin, hair tie, or silicone elastic band.**

7. **Repeat Steps 3 through 6 with the remaining sections of hair until your whole head is complete.**

TIP

When you unwrap your Bantu knots, you get another style that results in lovely curls you can rock for days. See Figure 10-8 for great examples of Bantu knots.

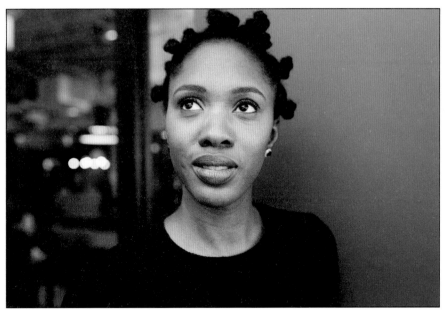

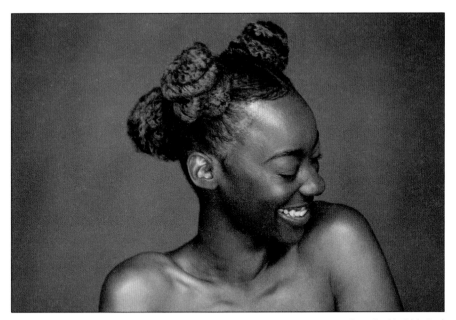

FIGURE 10-8:
Bantu knots,
big and small.

THE HISTORY OF BANTU KNOTS

Bantu knots are a traditional African hairstyle that have a long and sacred history. Historians have traced them back to the Zulu Kingdom in Africa. *Bantu* comes from the Zulu word for people, *Abantu. Abantu* originally referred to the hundreds of ethnic groups within southern Africa who spoke the Bantu language. When the Dutch colonized Southern Africa, they used the word "Bantu" as a derogatory name for the Zulu people. Eventually, the modern-day African diaspora reclaimed the word, and it's now used to reclaim the ancestral origins of the style.

Like I talk about throughout this book, many African cultures and people consider hair to be powerful and uniquely spiritual because it's the highest part of our bodies and closest to the heavens. Because of this, Bantu knots and other "high" styles are especially powerful and sacred. Bantu knots are a style that convey a true sense of pride and history, calling to mind the lives, struggles, and victories of the ancestors.

Shaping and Styling Afros

Letting your natural hair out unconstrained really is the easiest way to style your hair. You don't have to deal with braiding, twisting, or stretching — just let your hair *do what it do.* You don't need a whole lot of tools or time to style an afro, either. Don't get me wrong, crafting the perfect afro is a true art, but sometimes it feels nice to not have to use all of the other accoutrements. Afros are typically one specific look from the '70s, where your hair is fully picked out. But you may also see some people who do a wash-and-go on it without letting it get all puffy (see Figure 10-9). Either is fine; you rock what you like.

There are two main ways to start an afro, as shown in Figure 10-10:

>> You did a big chop, cutting your chemically treated hair off at the natural hair point.

>> You already have short hair.

To get your afro shaped, I highly recommend going to a professional barber. They have training and know exactly how to get your hair looking great and how to keep it healthy. You can go back in to get it reshaped about every two weeks.

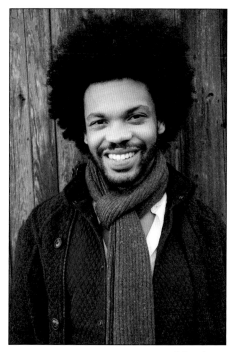

© Getty Images

FIGURE 10-9: Rocking an afro that's not fully picked out.

Daily styling of an afro involves only shaping it with your hands, following these steps:

1. **Start with dry clean hair.**

2. **Pick your hair thoroughly with a hair pick from root to tip.**

3. **Spray shine spray on it to keep it shiny and hydrated.**

4. **Lightly pat your afro to tweak the final shape.**

TIP

While your hair gets longer, it can get more tangled. Use a pick, along with a detangler and conditioner, to help gently detangle it every night. If you need a refresher on detangling, turn back to Chapter 4.

To maintain an afro, most importantly, keep your hair well hydrated and moisturized. Use a leave-in conditioner and oil (for help with choosing the right products, turn back to Chapter 7). While your hair grows, you can help it stay healthy by drinking a lot of water, eating hydrating foods, and shaping (or trimming) your hair periodically.

REMEMBER

When you get up in the morning, you may have to pick your afro, because it may be flat on one side. You may have heard that somewhere before, and that's good, because it's a legit reminder that as part of your morning afro care routine, you need to pick it out and reshape it after a night of sleeping on it.

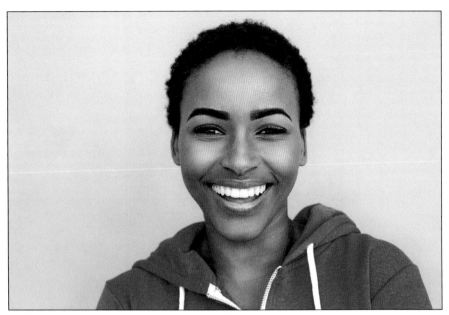

FIGURE 10-10:
Start your
natural hair
journey with a
short afro.

© mimagephotos/Adobe Stock

If you want to try afro puffs, divide your hair into two ponytails first, and then follow the same steps.

Building a Bun

Whether you're going for a casual or elegant look, wearing your hair in a bun helps you keep it protected. You can rock a messy bun on the weekend if you just need to go out and run some errands without having to fuss with your hair. Or you can elevate the look by styling a sleek bun for a night out.

If you want to know the truth, the easiest way to do a bun is probably with a bun sock or bun donut (I talk all about those tools in Chapter 12. Yes, I know that chapter is for kids; but honestly, bun donuts are for all ages). If you want to try a bun without using a donut, follow these steps:

1. **Start with freshly washed hair or use a spray bottle to dampen your hair.**

2. **Using a paddle or boar bristle brush, brush your hair.**

3. **Pull your hair in a ponytail in the location where you want the bun.**

4. **Apply gel to your hair to make it smooth.**

5. Divide your ponytail into two sections.

6. Twist the sections around each other.

7. Wrap the twisted ponytail around the base of ponytail and continue until all hair is wrapped.

8. Tuck the end into the bun wherever it lands.

9. Secure with bobby pins or hair pins.

10. Spray the bun with holding spray.

    Step 11 is optional.

11. Add edge control to style your hair line how you like.

The bun is as versatile as every other style. Stay simple or get creative. You can make it sleek, loose (like in Figure 10-11) or something in between! Do whatever feels right!

TIP

To get the bun look without using your own hair (or if you just want a bigger or more voluminous bun), buy a drawstring bun, which are synthetic buns that you can install by slipping onto a small knot or bun on your head and pulling the draw-strings closed. You can find them online or at beauty supply stores. You can also use extensions! Head over to YouTube to see videos of drawstring buns in action.

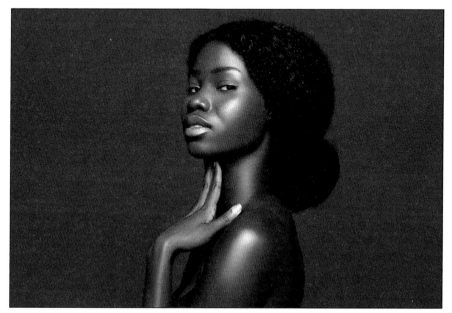

FIGURE 10-11:
A loose bun.

© Beauty Agent Studio/Adobe Stock

Using Scarves and Turbans

If you're looking for a stylish way to quickly get your hair up and off your face, a scarf or turban can do the trick. But I have to warn you: After you start using head wraps, you may become slightly addicted and soon have an entire collection in different colors and patterns.

WARNING

When using head wraps of any kind, make sure you don't wrap the fabric too tightly because it can give you a headache.

As often as possible, choose scarves and readymade turbans that are made of silk or satin because it reduces friction, but be sure to wear a wig cap underneath to keep them in place. If you want to wear a cotton head wrap, apply leave-in conditioner to your hair first to help keep it moisturized. Also consider wearing a silk- or satin-lined cap under a cotton head wrap to reduce friction.

Basic wrap

You can find countless ways to wear a head scarf. Follow these steps to start with one basic wrap:

1. **Position your scarf centered on your forehead.**
2. **Bring both ends to the back of your head and cross one side over the other.**
3. **Bring both ends to the front and tie them into a knot.**
4. **Twist the ends of your wrap together.**
5. **Bring both ends behind your head again, back to the front, and tuck the ends into the front knot.**

Turban wrap

You can try a creating a turban with a long scarf, as shown in the Figure 10-12. Follow these steps:

1. **Gather your hair at the top of your head to put your hair in a pineapple.**

   Chapter 5 has the how-to on pineappling.

2. **Place a scarf behind your head and bring the ends forward and cross them over each other.**

3. Bring the ends around to the back and tie the two ends together.

4. Tuck in the ends in to hide them.

5. Take out the loose hair tie from your pineapple.

6. Position or fluff your hair as needed, and be on your way!

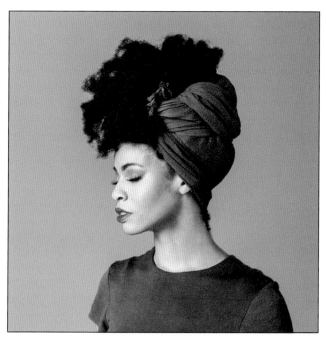

FIGURE 10-12: Create an updo using a scarf tied to contain your curls.

© Carlos David/Adobe Stock

5

Considerations for Kids

Uncover different characteristics of your child's hair and how it changes over time.

Manage your child's hair to keep it healthy.

Practice fun and easy kid-friendly styles.

Discover tips for creating a positive hair experience for you and your child.

IN THIS CHAPTER

» Getting to know your child's hair

» Helping your child embrace
their hair

» Introducing good hair habits to
your baby or child

» Advocating for your child's hair in
the community

Chapter **11**

Kiddie Curl Power

One of the main reasons I wrote this book is to help families. I'm here for parents, foster parents, aunties, uncles, friends, babysitters, and anyone who has a young person in their life.

If you're raising or caring for Black, Afro-Latinidad, biracial, or multiracial kids — especially if your hair texture and experience is different than theirs — you're probably looking for guidance. Let me be the first to welcome you with open arms and say, "You got this."

And let me just applaud and genuinely thank you for being here. Too many parents and guardians give up on their child's hair because it's too hard for them to care for. This type of rejection can do major damage to a child's self-esteem. It can make them feel insecure about their hair, like it's ugly or a burden. *So* many of my clients didn't start loving and embracing their naturally curly hair until well into their 20s because of their parents' negative energy, actions, and words about their hair. They grew up thinking they were less-than because their parents didn't take the time to figure out how to care for and love their hair like they could have. The fact that you're reading this book is an act of complete love and commitment to your child. Doing your child's hair builds a strong, positive foundation of trust, love, and mutual respect between you that can help shape your entire relationship.

This chapter can help you help your kids look and feel their best. It goes over the do's and don'ts of basic maintenance, starting from infancy and going through adolescence. And this chapter helps by giving you step-by-step styling options for your older child. I also show you how to act as your child's best hair advocate. Whatever your reason for reading this chapter, I'm here for it — and for you.

Understanding Your Child's Natural and Curly Hair

I'm here to help give you guidance for keeping your kids looking fresh, feeling fine, and celebrating who they are from their toes to their crown (see Figure 11-1).

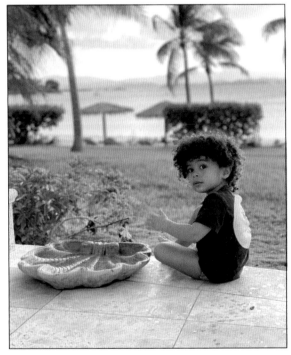

FIGURE 11-1:
Celebrate your child's hair every day, in every way.

Photo courtesy of Tamron Hall

Although I'm not a parent myself, I have a lot of kids in my life whom I care about. As a child's trusted adult and role model, you need to celebrate them as unique individuals and let them know they're beautiful and radiant. I am the positive, accomplished person that I am today because I believe I can walk through any door that I want to. I can figure out how to do what I need to do to get to where I want to go. Because growing up, my parents instilled a sense that I could do everything and anything I put my mind to. I could be and do anything I wanted.

I believed I could do anything because my parents believed it. The same is true of how I feel about doing hair.

Although you may find trying out new hair care skills frustrating at times, don't make the experience traumatic for your child. You, as the adult, can't take your own frustrations with trying to master a new skill out on your child.

Teaching your child to love and understand their natural hair starts the minute they're born (or the minute they join your life) and continues throughout their life. Set the stage for hair celebration by

>> Giving them dolls that have textured hair and the right hair tools so that they can practice on the dolls. The Fresh Dolls is a great line of dolls to check out.

>> Choosing books, TV shows, movies like "*Hair Love,*" and other media that feature characters who have natural and curly hair.

>> Taking them to salons or beauty shops that specialize in natural hair.

>> Filling their world with people who have textured hair.

>> Teaching them how to care for and style their hair (which is where I come in!).

TIP

If you want to add an extra dose of positivity, create an affirmation or mantra with or for your child. You can say it to them or with them as often as you like. You don't have to limit your affirmations to just hair, either. Any type of positive input you give to your child nurtures their whole self-image (see Figure 11-2).

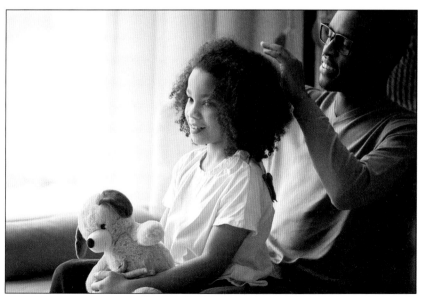

FIGURE 11-2: Incorporate positive words into your child's hair routine.

© Shutterstock.com

Thinking of Natural Hair as a Superpower

I would be remiss if I didn't acknowledge the struggle that people who have natural, textured hair have faced for centuries. From seeing natural hair portrayed in negative ways to not having the right tools and products easily available, to being pressured to relax natural curls — naturalistas have had to fight for society to view their hair as a positive attribute. The good news is, that fight is getting easier. I get that not everyone agrees with that statement, but I personally tend to lean positive and focus on what's working versus dwelling on what's not.

For an optimist like myself, understanding the stigma that the natural-and-curly-hair community has faced is an important piece of the puzzle — especially when it comes to kids. You should strive to understand that stigma (especially if that's not your experience) and do what you can to help overcome it. But you also have a choice in what to teach your kids about the past so that you can educate them, but also lift them up and instill pride in their hair (see Figure 11-3). To me, that means not setting them up to believe that everyone is against them and their hair.

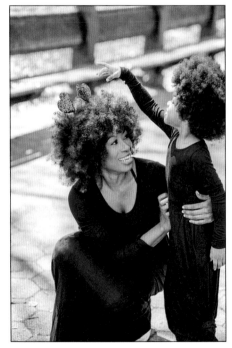

FIGURE 11-3: Teach your children to love their natural hair by example.

© Barbara Olsen/Pexels

So here's my hot take: You have a responsibility to teach them their cultural history, including the bits about hair, and the good and bad — while not damaging their future.

To help you and your child grow more in love with their hair, you can refer to Chapters 2 and 9 for some general guidance on natural hair care and styling. Beyond hair care, here are some ideas to provide your child with some positive reinforcement about their hair. Tell them

>> How textured hairstyles are highlighted, celebrated, and (let's be real) copied more than ever before.

>> About the beauty of their natural state.

>> Many natural styles have centuries of royalty and power behind them. In Chapter 9, I highlight some interesting historical facts about natural hair. Flip back there to learn more.

>> To honor their hair and care for it with love and respect.

Don't ignore their hair or the haters. Teach them how to celebrate their curls and to tell any meanies, "My hair is my superpower!"

TIP

If you carry unresolved trauma about your own hair, work to heal that trauma through individual therapy, support groups, or other counseling so that you can act as a role model to fully support your child's love of their hair.

Practicing Healthy Hair Habits from the Start

Your baby is born with hair (or maybe they come out a cue ball). Whatever they're born with, it changes while they grow. In the early years, help them create good general habits and hygiene through role modeling and letting them practice the hygiene as much as possible. Every kid is different, but I believe the more you allow them to try things for themselves, the more easily they can figure things out. Even toddlers can hold basic hair tools and mimic the movements of styling.

Throughout infancy, and even into toddlerhood for some (see Figure 11-4), follow a few basic best practices to get your child set up for hair-raising success:

>> Start with good healthy hair habits immediately by setting up a routine that they can follow throughout their life.

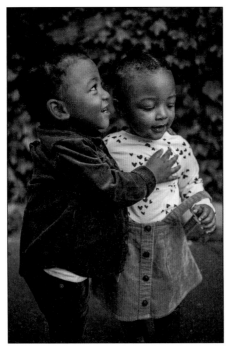

FIGURE 11-4:
Start healthy
hair habits with
young children
to lay a good
foundation
for life.

© Nina Hill/Unsplash

>> Your child's scalp is much more sensitive than your world-hardened adult head, so go easy on them. Some kids have sensitive scalps for a long time, even up to 4 or 5 years old.

WARNING

Watch out for the soft spot on the top of your baby's head! Always be cognizant of it and never apply pressure to that area because you could damage their skull or brain.

>> If your hair is a different texture than their hair, you need to care for their hair differently than you do your own.

>> Don't wash your child's curly hair every day. Curly hair doesn't get as oily as straighter hair, and curls dry out if you over-wash them. Wash their hair once a week, using a mild baby shampoo, if your kid has very tight coils. If they have looser curls, you can wash those curls two to three times per week, but only if you absolutely have to.

>> Between washes, you can co-wash their hair. Visit Chapter 4 for the how-to on co-washing.

>> At first, when your baby doesn't have much hair, their wash day doesn't take long. But while their hair grows, so does their wash-day routine. Expect the entire process to take awhile. Detangling can make the washing process feel

long, but protective styles can help keep tangles to a minimum. Visit Chapter 12 for ideas on those styles. Chapter 4 gives you the details on what to do during wash day. The only difference for kids: Make sure that you use kid-safe products that don't have parabens, fragrance, formaldehyde, dyes, or alcohol-based cleansers. Look at all labels before you buy!

» Comb your child's hair only when it's wet or it has conditioner on it. Never try to comb out textured hair when it's dry because it can break very easily.

» Use only wide-tooth combs on your child's curly hair when you're detangling. Fine-tooth combs can pull and break their hair. You can use detangling brushes, which are most often coated plastic and wide-toothed. Also, you can try using soft bristle brushes to better infuse conditioners into the cuticle, which reduces frizz after you rinse.

WARNING

Ideally, you should never use a hair accessory on a baby because accessories can damage their delicate follicles. Also, a baby might try to swallow an accessory. But if you want to use a simple headband, make sure it's completely soft materials and doesn't fit too tightly! Hard or tight accessories can damage their skull, fragile hair, and scalp permanently (not to mention, cause them discomfort and even pain). Accessories made with silk or satin may be better than cotton on curly hair. Cotton tends to be very absorbent and may contribute to loss of natural moisture or oils in the hair.

CARING FOR BIRACIAL OR MULTIRACIAL HAIR

If your child is biracial or multiracial, their hair may require different care techniques, products, and tools than what you may use for your own hair. If you don't have natural or curly hair yourself, you might struggle at first to figure out how to properly care for a hair texture different from your own. Once you practice some basic styling techniques, you'll gain skills and confidence. Plus, eventually, you can teach your kids to care for their own hair while they grow older!

If your child is multiracial, their hair might be different from strand to strand. In other words, they may have multiple hair types and textures on their head. I go more into detail about this mixture back in Chapter 3, if you want to read more.

When caring for a child that has multiple hair types, be sure to spend a lot of time with your child's unique head of hair. Keep an open mind and give yourself (and your child) plenty of grace and patience to get to know their hair and love it. If you're working on

(continued)

(continued)

new techniques that may challenge everything you know, that's okay. Remember that what works for one child might not work for another. And what works one day may not work the next. Allow experimentation — and most of all, don't give up! Keep practicing until you find what works best for your child. Caring for natural hair can be a beautiful experience for you and your child (see the accompanying photo)!

Also, if you personally don't have textured hair, you may not have experienced the trauma that can come from having your hair (or any part of you) degraded. Many adults who have textured hair have experienced this unhealed trauma and still contend with it to this day.

So many folks have grown up not having families who appreciate and care for every part of them. If you want to raise positive, self-aware kids who have high self-esteem, you have to love and nurture them as they are and not focus on how they're different from other family members. When you love your child fully, they love themselves fully.

The fact that you're reading this book tells me you're making a choice to see your child as the beautiful individual they are and not a complicated hair problem to solve. You can make this choice every day to not make their hair texture this overblown or overanalyzed thing. They're a complete and beautiful person — that's it and that's all.

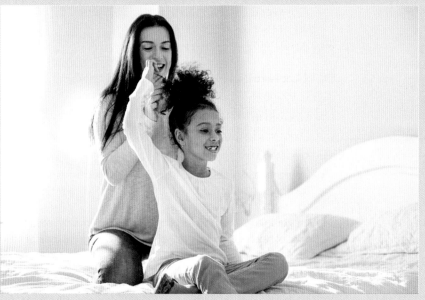

© Viacheslav Yakobchuk/Adobe Stock

Changes in curl type and texture

When your child is a baby, keep in mind that their hair is often softer, looser (maybe even straight), and more delicate than when they get older. When they're this young, you don't have to worry so much about their exact hair type and texture, but while they age, their hair texture most likely changes. You can check in on their type and texture (visit Chapter 3 on how to determine hair type and density).

Caring for your child's hair

If your child has a lot of hair, they need more help when it comes to washing, styling, and maintenance. At this point, the work starts to get serious. To begin to help yourself help your child, you do need to have a few basic ideas and skills under your belt, as discussed in the following sections.

Wash-day basics

Wash day can be challenging for kids and their parents because it can take up to several hours. Sitting or lying still for hours while their parents detangle, wash, condition, comb, and dry their hair can be very hard for children. And trying to keep a child calm and still during the wash-day process can be difficult for parents. I go over the step-by-step of how to wash and conditioner hair in Chapter 4, but here are some specific tips for making your child's wash day fun and successful for you both:

>> Create a routine. Kids thrive on structure and routine, so pick one day a week to do their wash day, and stick to it.

>> Talk with them about what they would like to add to the experience to make it their own. Do they want to listen to certain music? Maybe watch a special show on a tablet or phone?

>> Let your child help decide where they are most comfortable getting their hair detangled and washed, and in what position. That might mean lying on the kitchen or bathroom counter by the sink. It could mean sitting in a bathtub (either in a chair or right in the tub itself), or it could mean leaning over a sink or tub. And keep in mind, they might want to be in one position while detangling and another position for washing and conditioning. Together, you can find what works best for you and your child.

>> Wrap your child in a towel around their neck and shoulders to help catch water or product that may drip throughout the process, and have extra towels on hand to wipe their face as needed.

>> Make up special songs or games you can play during each step.

>> Let them participate as much as they can. That could mean letting them pick out their favorite comb or hair ties, helping to comb or detangle, or picking a towel to use to blot out the excess water at the end.

>> Use the time to tell secrets to each other. Share special stories or insights with your child, and invite them to do the same so it becomes a bonding time.

>> Set up a treat or reward system for wash day, if needed.

Daily care

Your child's hair requires care on the daily (the days that aren't wash days, anyway, which I talk about in the preceding section). Kids are very active, and even if they have tight or compressed styles, you will probably still have to style or care for their hair every day to some degree. You may not need to do this if their style is intact when they wake up, but if it's not, follow these steps in the morning to get your child's hair ready for the day:

1. **Spray a little water on your child's hair.**

   Make the hair slightly damp, not soaking wet.

2. **Divide the hair into sections if necessary, keeping the hair separated with duckbill clips or hair ties.**

   Steps 3 and 4 are optional.

3. **Rub a small amount of leave-in conditioner between your hands, and then gently rake it through each section or smoothing over the top of their strands from root to tip.**

   See Chapter 12 for a list of kid-friendly products.

4. **If your child's hair feels dry, apply a little oil or cream of your choice by using the technique described in Step 3.**

   Coconut oil is very popular. If you need help selecting an oil, visit Chapter 7.

5. **Style your child's hair (see Figure 11-5).**

REMEMBER

Babies and young children are much more sensitive than adults. Whenever you use any products, use as small an amount as you can get away with and watch closely for any rashes or signs of allergic reactions. If you notice anything unusual or alarming, stop using the product immediately and seek medical attention if needed.

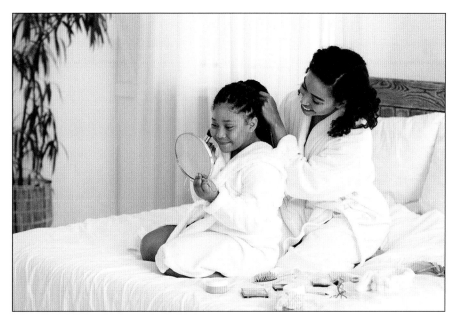

FIGURE 11-5:
Styling your
child's hair
provides an
opportunity for
some one-on-
one time.

© Prostock-studio/Adobe Stock

Styling your child's hair

The first step of styling your child's hair is to use the LOC (liquid, oil, and cream) method, as described in Chapter 6 to keep your child's hair healthy. Kids who have Type 4a to 4c high-porosity hair (as defined in Chapter 2) especially need the hydration that comes from the LOC method (see Chapter 4 for more information).

Although you can style your child's hair every day, many protective styles can stay in for a couple of weeks at a time. It's all about honoring your child's personal comfort and style. Many parents find wash-and-go's the easiest style to manage (see Figure 11-6), but for good hair health, help your child use protective styling regularly. You can apply some protective styles easily and relatively quickly, but others require far more labor and time such as the cornrows shown in Figure 11-6.

Start slow when they're young so that you both can get used to it together. If you have a younger child, you both may need extra patience. As time goes by, your child will learn to have patience. Don't worry, you both will be able to last longer and longer through the process. Refer back to Chapter 9 for a full rundown of all kinds of styles, such as braids, twists, and locs. And go to Chapter 12 for guidance on kid-friendly styles. When you feel ready, choose a style that you both want to try and just give it a go.

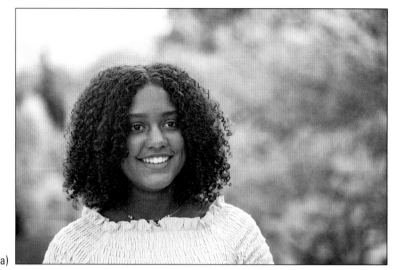

(a)

FIGURE 11-6:
Teens can style their own wash-and-go's (a), but other styles might require the help of a stylist (b).

(b)

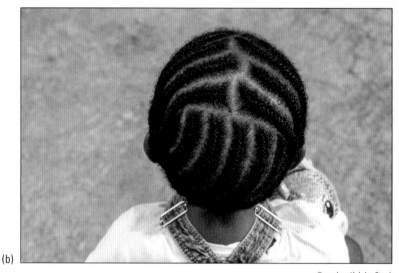

Always use silicone elastic bands or fabric-covered bands, shown in Figure 11-7, when styling your child's hair. Never use rubber bands because they can damage or break hair. And when you do use any type of hair ties, always remove them before bedtime because they can cause extra friction and tension on the hair, leading to breakage.

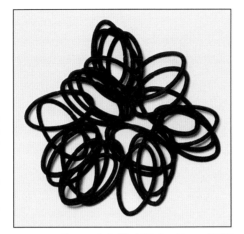

FIGURE 11-7:
Use silicone elastic or fabric-covered bands instead of rubber bands to avoid damaging your child's hair.

Photography by Wardell Malloy with crowdMGMT

WARNING

Never, ever do tight braids. Braiding your child's hair too tightly can cause traction alopecia (TA). Although it's reversible if you catch it in time, it's a very serious condition. I talk more about TA in Chapter 9, but suffice it to say, do everything you can to prevent it from happening in the first place.

If your child wants to experiment with non-protective styles, such as getting blowouts or having their hair straightened using a hot comb, let them. But let me just say, you can do these styles in the wrong way, and you can do them in the right way. *Hint:* The wrong way involves you doing it yourself. Nothing personal. Just promise to never, ever do it yourself, *mmmkay*? Leave anything involving heat, chemicals, or sharp tools to a pro. Need help finding a professional? Shimmy on over to Chapter 6 for some guidance.

TIP

Speaking of professional hairstylists, surround yourself with them! Feel no shame for playing the pro-help game. Be active in your own education and get the resources you need. Find a stylists (or several) who best understands and works with textured hair. Some stylists will even offer classes and courses that can show you how to care for and style natural and curly hair, especially if that isn't your own hair texture. Find out all you can, and then practice, practice, practice! And when you take your child into the salon, select hairstylists who are extremely patient with kids and newcomers, and who have an interest in helping people figure out how to embrace their natural hair.

If your child is rocking an afro (see Figure 11-8), afro puffs, or wash-and-go, you need to detangle and comb it regularly. Use a wide-tooth comb or pick, and go slowly.

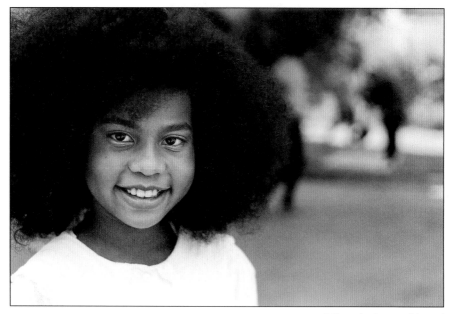

FIGURE 11-8:
Detangle
your child's
afro regularly
to keep it
healthy and
tangle-free.

Advocating for Natural Hair

Even though society seems to welcome natural, curly, and textured hair more than ever these days, you still have to keep your eyes open for unfair and unjust rules, particularly in schools, athletic events, and other regulated environments.

Many school districts still have rules against natural hairstyles, and you need to act as your child's number one advocate. Maybe you can thoroughly review the school handbook and call out racist or unjust policies, fighting to have those policies changed. Or maybe arrange a meeting with teachers, principals, or the school board to fight for your child's right to wear their hair however they please, just like everyone else. If nothing you do can make the district less biased, you may even choose to relocate your child to a district that's equitable in its policies.

Whatever your advocacy ends up looking like, the most important thing you can do is always be there for your child.

Chapter **12**

Kid-Friendly Styles and Products

I f you're having trouble figuring out how to style your child's hair, this chapter can help. Or maybe you're already a pro at a couple of styles, but you want to try some new ones. This chapter can help you, too. If you just need a crash course on which products to use and how, you've come to the right place.

Whether you're a complete newbie to the world of natural and curly hair or you're an old pro, this chapter walks you through how to give your child a style that's all their own.

Yes, figuring out your child's hair and style might take some practice and a lot of patience, but stick with it. Remember that helping your child express themselves through their hair is a fun and empowering experience. Flip through and read this chapter together. Look at the photos. Talk it over with them and let them select the style that speaks to them.

In this chapter, I take you through how to detangle before you start styling — a key first step in all great hairstyles. Then, you get to the super fun part — choosing a style. In this chapter, I give you a few ideas, but I encourage you and your child to make up your own designs and styles. Hair is so fun! Finally, I give you some guidance about kid-friendly products.

Setting the Stage for Styling Success

If styling your child's hair seems beyond your skill level, don't fret. Just be patient, move in small steps, and enjoy the learning process. Your child's hairstyle doesn't have to be perfect. In fact, the perfect hairstyle doesn't exist. Make the main goal having a fun and positive experience for both of you.

The beauty salon is such a cornerstone of the Black community for a reason — it provides a space to come together, catch up with each other, and look good for the day or week ahead. If you do want to bring your child to a salon when you need professional styling, choose a place and stylist who's experienced with kids. Look for someone who's patient, kind, engaging, and works well with them.

When doing your child's hair at home, you both can have the same experience as a salon but on a smaller scale, if you want it. Granted, you may not find doing your child's hair as easy as a pro would, and you might have a marked lack of gossip about what really went down at that barbeque after church last weekend.

REMEMBER

Each child's hair is different. Between genetics, environment, activity level, and personal style, your child has a mix that is truly all their own. Plus, your child's hair texture might change over time. Expect to do a lot of experimentation throughout their childhood.

Detangling Before You Style

Before you style your child's textured hair in any way, detangle it first. Don't forget this major fundamental rule. Curly, natural, textured hair can tangle easily, and if you want your child's hair to stay healthy and look good, you must detangle each wash day. I'll be honest with you: Detangling is a time-consuming step, and many kids don't like it. But it's a vital part of their hair care and styling, and the more you embrace it, the more they will, too. In Chapter 11, I give you tips on how to help your child find a comfortable position and other ways of making the detangling process comfortable and fun for them.

WARNING

Children are fragile and impressionable, so take care that you don't make a beautiful experience a traumatic one. I have clients who have all kinds of memories of getting burnt with pressing combs and relaxers, or getting their hair pulled and yanked at for hours. Their body stores that trauma, and I see them flinch in my chair involuntarily. But it doesn't have to be that way. You can make your child's experience positive, and they can build upon that for their whole lives.

To detangle your child's hair, follow four basic steps: Soak it, section it, condition it, and comb it. For a detailed detangling step-by-step and all of the tools you need to do it, turn back to Chapter 4. I discuss more about styling products designed for children in the section "Styling with Kid-Friendly Products," later in this chapter.

Go slow and take breaks when you (or your child) need to. Plan for a detangling session to last at least 30 minutes. If your child has a lot of hair or that hair seems extremely tangled, or if you're just beginning to figure out how to detangle, allow for more time. You definitely don't want to rush this step.

TIP

You can use distraction to make the detangling process more tolerable and fun. Find a new or special toy your child can play with or a favorite program that they can watch during the detangling process to help them focus their attention away from the process and sit still a little longer.

Styling Ideas for Your Child

When you style your child's hair, you have two main goals: Keep your child's hair healthy and protected, and help them express themselves in a way that makes them feel happy, proud, and radiant.

REMEMBER

Textured hair can tangle easily. And when you're talking about kids — who are constantly in motion — that's even more true. Remember to periodically use protective styling (such as braids or twists) to keep your child's hair healthy. Please flip back to Chapter 9 if you want details on how protective styling can benefit natural and curly hair.

Everyone knows how great it feels when your hair makes you feel and look good. Kids get that same feeling (see Figure 12-1).

Wash-and-go's

A *wash-and-go* is about the simplest hairstyle that you can use, as shown in Figure 12-2. They're exactly what they sound like: You wash your child's hair, then apply a leave-in conditioner and your favorite styling product to help define and hold their curl. That's it! They can go out into the world with their hair wet, air-drying over the next few hours. Or you can dry it by using a hair appliance, either a blow-dryer that has a diffuser attachment or a hooded dryer.

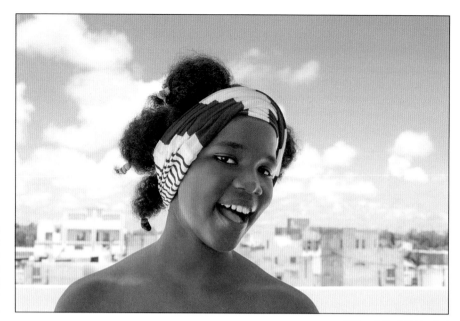

FIGURE 12-1:
Kids can create their own styles using scarves or other accessories.

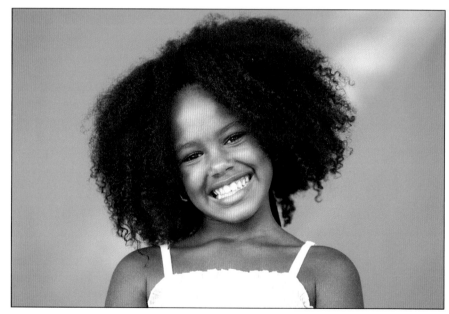

FIGURE 12-2:
A wash-and-go is a good option for kids who don't want to sit through a long styling process.

On very young children, use wash-and-go's almost exclusively. If your child is younger than 2 years old or has very little hair, they don't need much styling, so a wash-and-go is your best option.

TIP

Wash-and-go is also a great styling method for kids who just can't sit still very long, or if you're nervous at all about your styling skills. And giving your child a wash-and-go can help you to understand your child's hair texture. Just by having your hands in their strands, you can figure out so much about how it behaves and what it might need. Also, because it's so low-manipulation, it sets you and your child up to have a very positive, successful hair experience together to build upon in the future.

Although you don't have many steps to follow for a wash-and-go, if you prefer to see it laid out step by step, flip back to Chapter 9, where I give you a full play-by-play.

WARNING

Wash-and-go's can get more easily tangled on kids because they are always in motion, and they have their hands in their hair. This may mean you'll need to spend more time detangling.

Ponytails

After the wash-and-go, the second easiest way to style your child's hair involves giving them a ponytail or two. You don't need a lot of tools, and you don't have to know how to braid. And if you make a mistake or run into trouble, you can take out a ponytail pretty easily and start again.

However, if your child has a lot of hair, it can take a little more effort to gather that hair into a single ponytail. But overall, a ponytail gives you a good choice if you're looking for a basic first style to try.

REMEMBER

If your child likes to wear ponytails often, switch up the position from time to time to prevent too much wear and tear on their hair.

A ponytail is a great and easy style to use to keep your child's hair out of the way. Just remember that a lot of kids are too busy playing to keep their ponytail looking fresh all day, so you have to manage your expectations. You can start it out looking great, but by the end of the day, it might look a little messy. But it still does its job of keeping your child's hair back and out of their face while they live their busy lives.

You can start with dried wash day hair or daily detangled, moisturized hair (see Chapter 11). Then, follow these steps to give your kid a ponytail:

1. **Choose a location for the ponytail, and brush your child's hair using a boar bristle brush while gathering it all into your dominant hand.**

   Chapter 8 goes into your different brush options and why a boar bristle brush is the most effective choice for keeping hair smooth and put together without separating.

2. **Comb your child's hair using a rat tail comb to make it nice and smooth.**

3. **Once it's all smooth and flat, take your hair tie of choice and wrap it snugly (taut but not tight) around the hair.**

4. **To get the hair tie positioned even more snugly, separate the ponytail in two sections and pull lightly in separate directions so the hair tie slides down towards the skull.**

5. **You can use gel or pomade around the base of the ponytail and the hairline to finish the style and keep flyaways down.**

If you need to refresh your child's ponytail, you can re-wet it and then smooth in a bit of leave-in conditioner with your hands.

WARNING

Never use rubber bands on hair, particularly on textured hair. The rubber is porous and absorbs the moisture from the hair, leading to tangles, damage, and a lot of hair pulling, which could lead to traction alopecia over time. You should use silicone elastic bands or fabric-covered bands instead.

Twists and braids

I give the step-by-step instructions of all kinds of twists and braids in Chapter 9 but are shown in Figure 12-3. To braid or twist your child's hair, you can follow the exact same steps that appear in that chapter. If you braid your child's hair and happen to notice that their hair is breaking in braids, try two-strand twists instead. They tend to be gentler on the hair.

WARNING

This bears repeating — especially for children. Don't braid their hair too tightly. Over time, too-tight braids may damage their scalp from the tension, leading to hair loss due to traction alopecia. (I go into more detail on the dangers of braiding too tightly in Chapter 9, as well.)

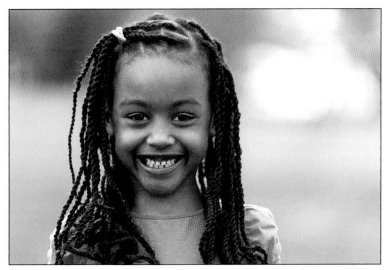

© Samuel Borges Photography/Shutterstock

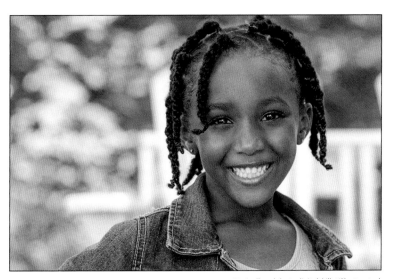

© pixelheadphoto digitalskillet/Shutterstock

Afros and puffs

Afros and afro puffs are fun and easy options for your child. An afro is super simple: Just allow natural growth to do its thing, loose and free. And afro puffs are basically an afro smoothed into a single updo or divided into two (or more) curly sections, called *puffs*.

ADDING BEADS

Your child may want to accessorize their braids with beads (as shown in the accompanying photo). Just don't use too many beads because they can add extra weight to the hair. The more weight on their hair, the more their hair gets pulled and damaged.

To add beads to your child's braid, you need a hair beader tool and large-hole hair beads. You can find these items at a beauty supply store. Ask for help in choosing one that is right for your child.

After you have your child's hair braided or twisted (which I describe in Chapter 9), follow these steps to add beads:

1. **Line up the beads that you want to put on the braid, in order.**

   The bead you put on the tool first will end up on the bottom of the braid.

2. **Put the braid through the beader loop.**

3. **Pull the braid through the beads.**

4. **Take the very end tip of the braid and wrap back up and tuck it into the last bead.**

5. **Wrap a tiny silicone elastic band around the hair just above that last bead to secure it.**

   The elastic band helps keep the beads in place.

Note: The instructions also work for adding beads to twists.

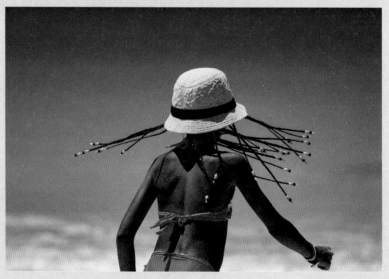

© laura/Adobe Stock

Follow these steps to style your child's afro, as shown in Figure 12-4:

1. **Spray your child's hair with water to get it damp (not dripping wet).**

   Make sure to spray the front, sides, and back of their head.

2. **Apply leave-in conditioner or oil from the root of their hair to the tip, covering the hair completely. If your child's hair is dense or thick, you may have to section it for this step.**

   The section "Styling with Kid-Friendly Products," later in this chapter, gives you some ideas for what types of conditioners or oil to use.

3. **Brush with a boar bristle brush back around the hairline.**

   Chapter 8 goes into the benefits of boar bristle brushes.

4. **Rub a small amount of gel onto your palms and smooth the hair back around their hairline.**

   Brush their hair with a soft toothbrush if you need extra help smoothing the hair.

   Step 5 is adding an optional accessory.

5. **Use an elastic headband or ribbon-like hair tie to contain and shape the afro.**

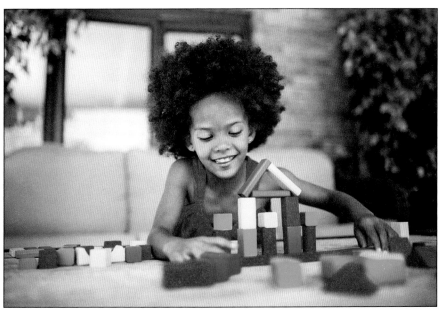

FIGURE 12-4:
A few steps is all it takes to style your child's afro.

© Getty Images

Here is how to use a headband or hair tie:

- *Headband:* Put the headband over their head and down on their neck, like a necklace. Then bring it up to their front hairline and push it up and over their ears. If the headband is too loose, twist it and wrap it around their hair once more.

- *Hair tie:* Wrap it around the back of their head and tie it in front — in a bow or decorative knot.

TIP

If you want to do a more protective style, you can tie a silk or satin scarf around their hairline or use a silk or satin-lined headband. If you go this route, use bobby pins to secure the scarf because it may slip because your child is so active.

If you want to try an afro puff, as shown in Figure 12-5, or puffs, follow the preceding instructions through Step 4. Then, follow these steps:

1. **Gather the hair into one high ponytail or two ponytails on either side of the head, using fabric-covered hair ties.**

2. **Shape the puff or puffs gently, using a pick and your hands.**

   Mold them into the puff shape you want.

3. **Mist the hair lightly if it starts to dry to help you shape the puffs.**

   Just don't oversaturate because it will be too wet to shape.

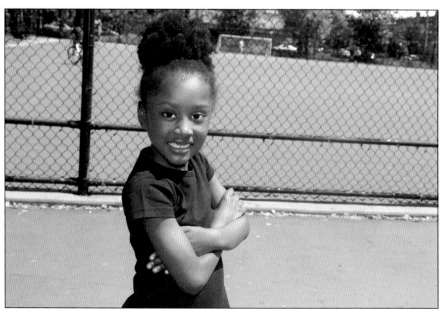

FIGURE 12-5:
A child with an afro puff.

Buns

Buns can keep hair up and out of the way (see Figure 12-6). The easiest way to give your child a bun is probably with a bun donut, which you can find at any local beauty supply or drugstore.

The bun donut looks like a spongy donut, and it comes in various colors so that it can blend in with hair. You can also DIY by cutting the top off a tube sock at home, but I don't recommend it because the donut gives you a near-perfect result every time, and it doesn't cost much at all. Using a sock is more challenging because it's looser and your bun may not come out as tightly and neat. For a few bucks, go get yourself one at the local drugstore. Most bun donuts come with instructions, but follow these basic steps to use one:

1. **Apply a bit of gel to your child's very moisturized hair.**

2. **Brush the hair with a boar bristle brush to gather it into a high or low ponytail.**

   Hold the hair in one hand.

3. **Push the hair through the bun donut.**

4. **Fold, wrap, and smooth your child's hair over the donut, tucking in all bits of hair.**

   Use hair pins if you need to secure any loose ends.

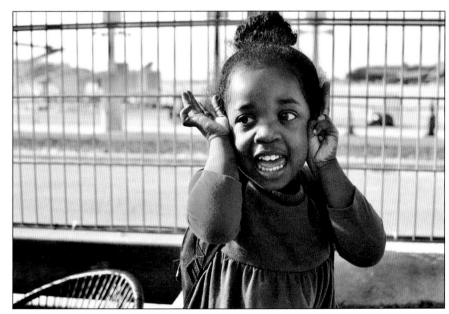

FIGURE 12-6: A bun keeps a child's hair out of the way of their busy hands.

© Ilona Virgin/Unsplash.com

If you don't want to use a bun donut, I offer another method in Chapter 10.

Mohawks

Okay, so if your child wants a mohawk, you probably need to take a trip to the barber or salon. That said, mohawks are possible for kids who have natural and curly hair are extremely popular right now. And mohawks have been a mark of the cool kids for decades. Mohawks look super fresh when done by the right professional, and your kid can work with the stylist to choose how fancy or unique they want it to look. Some options you can talk over with your stylist include

>> Curly hair mohawks — a wash-and-go cut into a mohawk shape where your curls are left out on top, but the sides are super short (see Figure 12-7).

>> Graphic mohawks — a mohawk where the stylist shaves designs into the side of your head.

>> Braided mohawks — your hair is braided flat on the sides with loose braids in the middle on top.

>> Faded undercut mohawks — the sides are shaved very close to the skin on the sides, and there's a fade under the hair on top.

>> Short mohawks — this is when your hair on top isn't very long, but is cut into a strip or mohawk, and is still is longer than the sides.

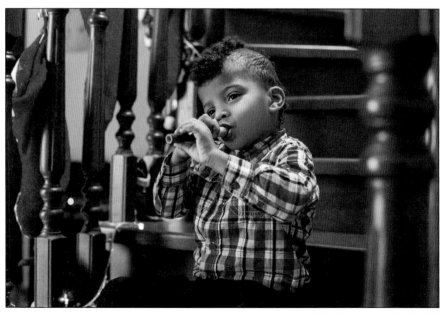

FIGURE 12-7:
A child with a
curly mohawk.

© DenisProduction.com/Adobe Stock

Styling with Kid-Friendly Products

I offer a complete rundown of what to look for in hair care and styling products in Chapter 7. Although my specific product recommendations are more geared towards adults, the information about ingredients, what to look for and stay away from, and even how to make or use your own natural hair products all apply to products for children, as well.

Here are some general tips for you when you're out there trying new products for your child. Keep in mind, they may be different from what works for you:

» Look for sulfate-free and paraben-free products.

» Select products that are marked as gentle and/or tear-free.

» Look for products that clearly boast ingredients that are vegan and gluten free if you have any allergy concerns.

» Ask for product recommendations from parents of other children who have textured hair.

Always let your child style or cut their hair however they want, no matter what your own opinion is. Remember that all hairstyles are temporary. Hair will grow back. Sometimes you might think they're going to end up hating their idea. So what? Resist the urge to stop them from trying. Let them try. If they hate it, well — now they know. But let them have fun while trying a different hairstyle.

6

The Part of Tens

Discover my do's and don'ts for keeping your curls cute.

Find your best look with tips from the pros.

Explore how you can become your own healthy hair advocate to celebrate your curls.

Chapter **13**

Ten Natural and Curly Hair Do's and Don'ts

L ove is in the hair, and no matter what you've read or heard in the past, attaining healthy natural and curly hair doesn't have to be difficult. Although you don't have to follow any rules on your natural hair journey, I can give you a few do's and don'ts that you can implement (or avoid) in your hair care regimen to help you achieve healthy hair.

In this chapter, I set you up with ten essential do's and don'ts for a successful healthy hair journey. If you read nothing else in this book, this chapter can help you start new habits that are easy enough to do, but are foundational enough to make big changes for your hair.

Do: Take Care of Your Scalp

A healthy scalp is the key to maintaining optimal hair health. Make sure your scalp stays clean and free of buildup by using these tips:

» Give yourself a daily scalp massage to help enhance blood circulation and stimulate hair growth. Hair growth starts at the roots, so you must create a healthy foundation.

» You can apply tea tree oil to your scalp. I wouldn't do it every day, but twice a week. (You can apply the oil while massaging your scalp, getting two things accomplished at the same time!) Take care to avoid scratching or pricking your head. If the tea tree oil gets in a scratch, it may cause irritation.

» Rinse your hair and scalp by using apple cider vinegar before shampooing and conditioning.

» Use a clarifying shampoo when you need to remove buildup. Follow up with your favorite moisturizing shampoo to normalize the hair and scalp pH.

For more how-tos and tips on caring for your scalp, flip back to Chapter 4.

Don't: Skip or Rush Detangling

Natural and curly hair definitely needs regular detangling. I know it can be tempting to skip it, but never do. Although skipping detangling might feel easier and like it's saving you time, it really causes you problems and costs way more time when you have to deal with the consequences later.

If you leave your hair tangled, it can mat and ultimately break, so just bite the bullet and embrace the detangling. That means also taking your time when you do it. Rushing the detangling process can create abrasions on your hair shaft.

Set aside enough time on wash day to ensure you can devote the time and attention this task needs. Be sure to detangle in small sections, starting at the ends and work your way up. Visit Chapter 4 for all the how-tos on detangling.

TIP

Find a way to make detangling more pleasant. Maybe *bump* some music or use a product that has your favorite fragrance. Whatever it is, find something that creates a fun and positive association for your detangling sessions.

Do: Steam Treat Your Curls

In a *steam treatment,* moist heat helps open the cuticle layer of your hair and the pores on your scalp to allow better absorption of your conditioners and treatments. Steam treatments enhance product absorption, improve elasticity and curl definition, and improve scalp health.

For more on steam treatments, go back to Chapter 4.

Don't: Neglect Your Split Ends

I know it sounds counterintuitive, but trimming your hair actually encourages hair growth. Split ends not only can cause damage to the rest of the hair shaft, they also make your hair look thin and make it more difficult to detangle.

Try not to obsess over your hair length. Instead, focus more on your hair's health by getting regular trims every two months or so. This schedule keeps your hair at its absolute best. If you neglect scheduling a trim every six to eight weeks, you just can't maintain truly healthy hair and see the benefits of all of the rest of your healthy hair regimen.

TIP

If you can't get a trim every two months, at least aim for the bare minimum of every six months.

Do: Protect Your Hair at Night

Good hair care is not just about what happens on wash day. Caring for your hair is a daily responsibility. Most people have at least a small morning hair routine so that they don't look a fright when they step out of the house. But I'm here to say that your nighttime routine does as much for keeping your hair looking great as your morning routine does. Don't skip it! Everyone's hair is different, so you have to figure out what works for you; but always protect your hair at night.

Before you go to sleep, cover your head with a satin or silk bonnet or scarf, or you can sleep on a satin or silk pillowcase. These materials help keep the moisture in your hair. It also reduces friction on your hair, which helps you maintain your curls and prevent frizz.

Don't: Heat Style Too Often

After working so hard to get your curls healthy, the last thing you want to do is ruin them with excessive heat. I know we all love a good blowout, and that's totally fine, but stick to doing it only every now and then, and always use a heat protectant. The same goes for using curling irons, flat irons, hot combs, or other heat tools. Constant heat styling can cause damage to your curls and leave them looking limp and over-stretched.

TIP

If you're currently using a lot of heat on your hair, it might take some time to break the heat habit. If you can't go cold turkey, that's okay. Try the opposite approach. Start by picking one day a week when you won't use heat. Then keep adding "no heat" days until you're using heat to style your hair for special occasions only.

Do: Deep Condition Regularly

If you're going to condition on wash day, why not deep condition? Deep conditioners can contain hydrating and strengthening agents such as protein, natural extracts, and oils that really enhance the overall health of your hair and assist with moisture retention. Deep conditioning can help prevent damage, improve elasticity, and enhance shine, among other things.

Here are a few tips for effective deep conditioning:

>> Before you apply your deep conditioner, squeeze or blot your hair with a towel to get rid of excess water. Removing excess water helps the conditioner further penetrate your hair strands.

>> Apply the conditioner from tip to root and leave it on 20 to 30 minutes or what the manufacturer's label indicates.

>> Use cool water to rinse the conditioner out to help seal your hair's *cuticle* (the outer layer).

Don't: Over-Manipulate Your Curls

Yes, you need to manipulate your hair to care for and maintain it, but don't over-manipulate it. Too much manipulation can cause your hair to break. When it comes to handling your hair, try not to touch it any more than necessary, and when you do have to touch it, be as gentle as possible.

REMEMBER

You can combat the hand-in-hair syndrome by wearing low-manipulation and protective styles from time to time. Buns, low or high ponytails, and pineapple puffs are all great low-manipulation options, but wearing them too tightly or too often can cause breakage around your entire hairline. You have to switch up your styling.

Do: Take Care of All of You

Your hair is part of a whole ecosystem. When one part of you is out of whack, your whole system can stop working like it should. So do whatever you can to take care of your mind and body. Beyond the tresses on your head, I recommend focusing on three main health and wellness goals to help your hair (and the rest of you) live its best life:

>> **Exercise regularly.** When you exercise, you increase your blood circulation. This increased circulation allows blood, nutrients, and oxygen to get to your scalp. This blood flow enhances your hair follicles, keeping them strong and healthy. Exercising also reduces stress, and we all know the effects stress has on our strands (looking at you, gray hair!).

>> **Maintain a balanced diet.** Eating right gives your follicles the nutrients needed to help your curls thrive. You are what you eat, and most of the time, when you can't figure out why you can't keep your hair healthy, remember that healthy hair starts from within. Eat foods such as fatty fish, eggs, leafy greens, berries, and nuts to see a big difference in your hair (and skin).

>> **Hydrate properly.** Water is the cornerstone of all life, including hair care. Your hair needs water more than anything else. Your shampoos, conditioners, oils, and other products help hydrate and moisturize your hair from the outside, but they're not enough. Every day, aim to drink about a half ounce to one ounce of water per pound that you weigh.

Don't: Skip or Delay Wash Day

The most basic thing you can do to care for your hair is to wash and condition it regularly. Resist the urge to delay or totally skip your wash-day routine. You need to clean your hair of buildup on a regular basis, especially if you use products regularly. But you don't need to over-wash it; once every seven to ten days is perfect. Rotate using clarifying shampoo with moisturizing shampoos. Using clarifiers every time you shampoo can unknowingly remove needed natural moisture from the hair. Create good habits for yourself until they become muscle memory. Wash your hair on the same day — at the same time, if you can. Being consistent with your wash days takes the mental workout out of it. No need to waste energy wondering when you can fit it into your schedule or how you can get yourself out of it. Just plan for it without debate. It makes the process smoother and your hair and scalp will thank you for it.

TIP

If wash days fill you with resistance, flip the script. Make the experience more fun by burning scented candles, playing music, eating good food afterwards — whatever brings you joy, add it to your wash-day routine.

Chapter **14**

Ten Hairstyling Tips from Industry Experts

I've been fortunate enough to work in the beauty industry for over 30 years now. After all these years, I'm still very passionate about hairstyling, and I find great joy in servicing and educating my clients and peers. Throughout the years, I've had the pleasure of connecting with some remarkable industry experts who share this same passion. I've worked with some of the folks whose tips I include in this chapter, and I've admired some from afar.

Although I consider myself an expert, the natural and curly hair movement has come such a long way since the beginning of my career, and it constantly evolves. I don't know it all (there's no way I could!), so I've asked my esteemed colleagues from across the U.S. to share their favorite natural or curly hair tips with you here. (That means you're getting natural and curly hair guidance from not one, but more than 11 hair professionals in this book. What a deal!)

The experts I rounded up for this chapter have amazing careers. I'm so honored to be able to include their words in this book. A few of the tips here back up some of the information I cover elsewhere in the book, and other tips reveal nuances and additional information that I don't cover. Some of these tips do cover the same topics, but from different angles. In the same way that everyone's hair is unique, every hairstylist has their own unique opinion based on their specific experiences. Whether these tips give you new insight, reinforce a fundamental lesson I share in other chapters, or offer an opposite take, they can definitely help you along your natural hair journey.

Combat Hair Loss with Keratin Fibers

This tip comes from Jacqueline Tarrant (see Figure 14-1), beauty expert, consultant, columnist, and owner of the Natural Hair Bar in Chicago, Illinois. You can visit Jacqueline at www.naturalhairbar.com or on Instagram at @thenaturalhairbar.

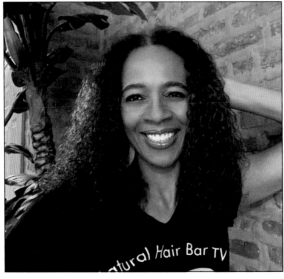

FIGURE 14-1: Jacqueline Tarrant, the expert behind Natural Hair Bar.

Photography by Charan Ingram

"More than 50 percent of women will experience noticeable hair loss in their lifetimes, and three out of five women are currently suffering from hair thinning. Those numbers may be shocking, but there is hope. There are many causes of hair loss. Sometimes genetics causes it. Other times, self-inflicted aggressive styling causes it, which leads to a condition known as traction alopecia. This type of hair loss can become permanent when repeated tension and friction causes the hair thinning to progress to scarring, ultimately causing irreversible hair loss.

"As a certified trichologist, I treat women of all ages who are suffering from hair loss. The best solution is to give your hair a rest from all tension-based styles, including braids, weaves, cornrows, tight ponytails, and even wigs (the rubbing of them against the head can cause hair loss). Begin a regular treatment regimen and allow your follicles to heal, and your hair will begin to regrow. During the regrowth process, you can use keratin powder to cover thinning hair. *Keratin powder* is made of hair-building keratin fibers that are nearly identical to human hair. These fibers blend naturally and bind undetectably to even fine hair.

"Here's how I treated one client, and it may work for others battling hair loss, too.

"Figure 14-2 shows how she looked when she came to me. We came up with a plan, and we turned it into a makeover. Here are the steps I took:

1. Shampooed, conditioned, and defined her curls, as you can see in Figure 14-3.

2. Applied clip-in curly tracks to blend with her natural curly hair, as you can see in Figure 14-4.

3. Sprinkled keratin fibers that matched her hair color to cover and blend into thinning area, as seen in Figure 14-5.

"Voila! Confidence restored (see Figure 14-6)."

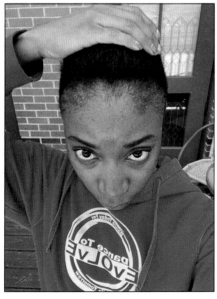

FIGURE 14-2: Alexis was ready for a change after dealing with hair loss.

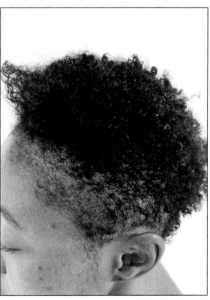

Photography by Charan Ingram

Photography by Charan Ingram

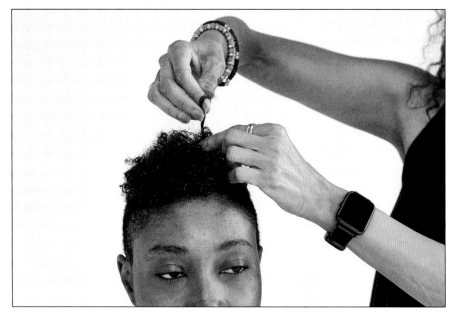

FIGURE 14-3:
Defining Alexis'
curls.

Photography by Charan Ingram

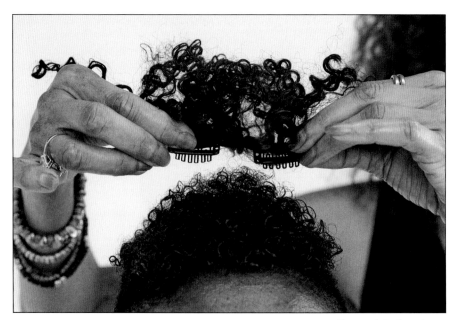

FIGURE 14-4:
Applying
matching clip-
in tracks.

Photography by Charan Ingram

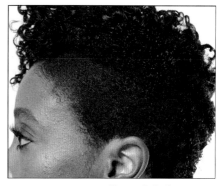

FIGURE 14-5: Keratin fibers can help in the hair loss recovery process.

Photography by Charan Ingram

Photography by Charan Ingram

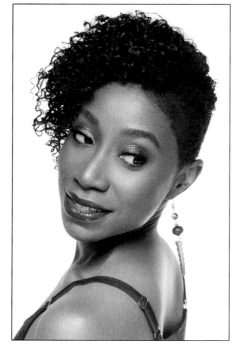

FIGURE 14-6: The finished look.

Photography by Charan Ingram

Stop Double Conditioning

Monica Stevens (shown in Figure 14-7) — licensed cosmetologist, content creator, Sally Beauty texture stylist, Aveda Texture Team member, and founder of the MoKnowsHair Curl Collection product line — shares the following tip. You can find Mo at www.moknowshair.com and on YouTube, Instagram, Facebook, and Twitter as @MoKnowsHair.

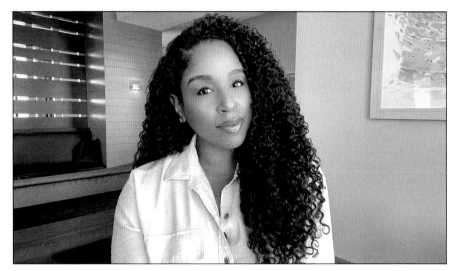

FIGURE 14-7: Monica Stevens, the expert behind MoKnowsHair Curl Collection.

"Do you have super frizzy, barely-there curls that won't hold style and feel like straw, even though you frequently use *two* conditioners on wash day? If you're using a rinse-out (daily) conditioner and deep conditioner (mask/treatment) in the same wash day routine, you're wasting your time and product. On wash day, pick one or the other, not both!

"After shampooing, if you apply a rinse-out conditioner (surface conditioners made to protect, smooth, or hydrate for one to three days), your pH lowers and the conditioner attaches to the outside of your strands. Your deep conditioner (formulated with lower molecular weight, allowing it to penetrate strands with lasting effects of repair and hydration for four to seven days, on average) has a lower pH than shampoo, so it will sit on top of your rinse-out conditioner and next to nothing happens; you're not getting the benefits of the treatment because your strands are already covered by the first conditioner you applied. You are essentially wasting your time and your money as you rinse your deep treatment down the drain."

Treat Your Twist Outs Well

This tip is courtesy of celebrity hairstylist and entrepreneur Larry J. Sims (shown in Figure 14-8). You can find Larry on Instagram at @larryjarahsims.

"I LOVE TEXTURE. The most versatile textures, in my opinion, are 4a to 4c. They allow you to create texture and shape within their original texture in a beautiful way.

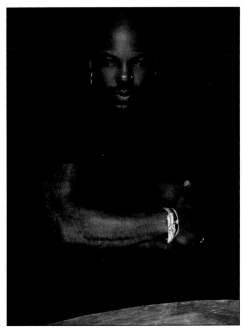

FIGURE 14-8:
Celebrity
hairstylist and
entrepreneur
Larry J. Sims.

Photography by Dae Howerton

"Elongated twist outs are one of my favorite styles for these textures. My go-to tip to maximize the stretch in your twist outs is to blow dry your hair with a Denman/paddle brush to a smooth finish.

"Also, I LOVE using Flawless By Gabrielle Union Curl Cream to set my twist outs, especially on hair that's been pre-stretched with a blowout. It provides a soft, elongated, and moisturized finish." For more on pre-stretching, visit Chapter 9.

Use Leave-In Conditioner to Seal Your Hair's Cuticle

Celebrity hairstylist, artistic director, and spokesperson Tippi Shorter Rank's work has appeared in *Vanity Fair, O, Essence,* and others. (See this hairstyle maven in Figure 14-9.) You can find Tippi on Instagram at @tippishorter and visit her at www.tippishorter.com. She gives the following advice about natural and curly hair care.

"My favorite tip to share is about prepping hair and making sure your unique fabric [hair] is balanced and ready to receive your styling products. You can prep your hair to receive your styling products by using a leave-in conditioner.

It softens hair, makes detangling easy, balances the pH, restores moisture, seals the cuticle, and so much more. One way to ensure your leave-in (or other prep product) is sealing cuticles and easing the tangles is to keep it in the refrigerator. When you apply anything that is cool (your conditioner, other products, or even water or air) to your hair, you help seal your hair's cuticle. A sealed cuticle reduces tangles, keeps hair shiny, makes strands feel smoother, and allows styling product to perform better and last longer."

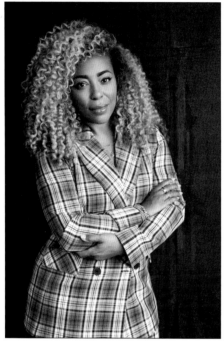

FIGURE 14-9:
Celebrity hairstylist Tippi Shorter Rank.

Photography by Carlisha Nunnally

Detangle Regularly

Evie Johnson (shown in Figure 14-10) — certified trichologist, salon owner, platform stylist, and educator — shares this tip. You can find Evie at www.eviejohnsonclasses.com and on Instagram at @contactevie.

"One of my favorite tips for curly or natural hair is to detangle, and keep your hair hydrated according to your texture types at all times.

"And here's a bonus for you: I absolutely love to do two-strand twists to help with elongation of coils or curls."

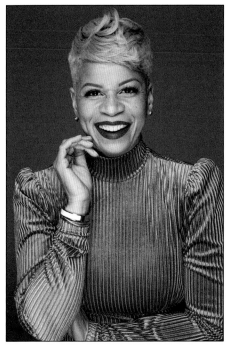

FIGURE 14-10:
Certified
trichologist,
salon owner,
platform stylist,
and educator
Evie Johnson.

Photography by Renny Vasquez

Master the Wash-and-Go

This tip comes from New York-based Ursula Stephen (see Figure 14-11), celebrity hairstylist and New Image Beauty Expert. You can find Ursula at www. ursulastephenthesalon.com and on Instagram at @ursulastephen.

"My fave tip for styling curly and natural hair is a combination of a few tips for getting a great wash-and-go:

>> During the conditioning step of the shampoo process, I always recommend detangling the hair. This makes styling (and life) easier for me.

>> When you add leave-in conditioner to your hair, make sure it is soaking wet. Never let that hair dry before adding products!

>> Apply leave-in conditioner from root to tip, while raking your fingers through your hair. This distributes the products while detangling.

>> After conditioning and detangling, squeeze your hair to release excess product and water.

>> Apply your favorite styling cream in medium sections.

>> Allow your hair to air dry for a moment, then follow with a diffuser for a fluffy, and sexy wash-and-go."

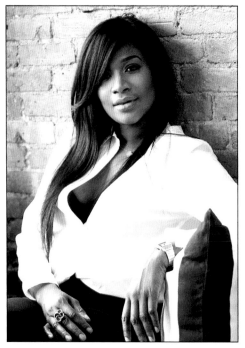

FIGURE 14-11:
Celebrity
hairstylist
and New
Image Beauty
Expert Ursula
Stephen.

Photo courtesy of Ursula Stephen

Add Extra Love to Your Protective Styles

Nicole Mangrum, in Figure 14-12, is a Chicago native and renowned hairstylist, artist, and entrepreneur. Her 25-plus years of work as a hair artist has earned her three Make-Up Artists & Hair Stylists (MUAHS) Guild award nominations. You can find Nicole on all social media at @nicolemangrumhair and visit her at www.nicolemangrum.com. She offers this advice.

"As a natural hair enthusiast and wig–rocking curly girl, I love wearing wigs as a protective style to add versatility to my looks, protect my hair, and encourage growth. A protective hairstyle could also be braids, twists, an updo, or locs that don't require much maintenance or daily manipulation of the hair.

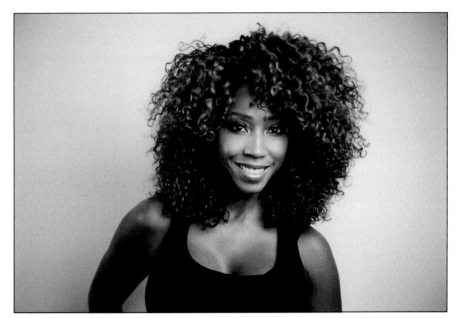

FIGURE 14-12:
Renown
hairstylist and
entrepreneur
Nicole
Mangrum.

Photography by Billy Rood

"Before putting your hair in a wig or any protective style, give it some extra love by prepping it with a clarifying shampoo, fortifying treatment, and deep conditioning masque. Lastly, add coconut or olive oil to seal in the moisture.

"Here are a few more quick but important tips about protecting your natural hair:

>> Don't forget about your hair and scalp underneath. Cleanse and condition once a week, depending on the protective style. I like to use an applicator bottle to apply shampoo diluted with a bit of water, plus a few drops of tea tree oil and really get under my braids. Lather, rinse thoroughly, and spray on a liquid leave-in conditioner for extra hydration. Dry completely.

>> Never sleep with wet hair. Make sure to dry braids by sitting under a hooded dryer or using a hairdryer to remove the water before sleeping to prevent bacteria and odor from developing.

>> Be sure that the braids under your wig aren't too tight, and utilize a stocking cap to prevent friction and breakage along the hairline."

Hydrate, Trim, and Have Fun

Tym Wallace (shown in Figure 14-13), celebrity hairstylist and makeup artist, offers three tips in one. You can find Tym on Instagram at @tymwallacehair.

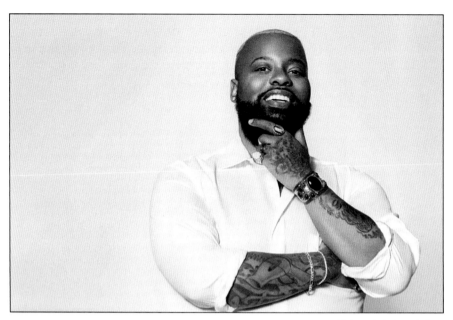

FIGURE 14-13:
Tym Wallace, celebrity hairstylist and makeup artist.

Photography by James Anthony

"My go-to tip for natural hair is to, number one, make sure you keep it hydrated! Moisture, moisture, moisture is good for natural hair. Remember, a good moisture-protein balance is important for giving your hair more vibrancy.

"Secondly, I believe in keeping your ends trimmed every six to eight weeks. A good trim will always keep your hair healthy.

"Lastly, have fun! There are so many fun ways to style your hair, from Bantu knots, to cornrows, to faux braids and locs, to all types of fun ponytails and so many textured styles. The sky is the limit! Our hair defies gravity!"

Use Steam to Improve Absorption

Chicago-based celebrity hairstylist, beauty expert, and entrepreneur Kim Kimble (see Figure 14-14) shares this tip. You can visit Kim at www.shopkimkimble. com, on Instagram and Twitter at @kimblehaircare, and on Facebook at @ kimblehairstudio.

"When it comes to natural hair care, products that are made to hydrate and moisturize are key. They usually work well for styling and maintaining curly hair on their own, but some natural hair has low porosity, which means that your hair doesn't absorb products well. One way to help improve this issue is to first make sure your conditioners, hair masks, and oils are very rich in hydration. Before you apply them, use a heating cap (it uses direct heat to generate steam) or steamer to help open your hair's cuticle, which softens your hair and makes sure the products penetrate your hair.

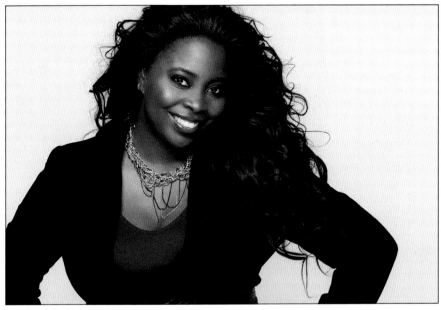

FIGURE 14-14:
Celebrity hairstylist, beauty expert, and entrepreneur Kim Kimble.

Photography by Dandre Michael

"Last but not least, always sleep with a silk bonnet, pillowcase, or scarf because cotton dries out your hair. The silk keeps hair soft, silky, and hydrated."

Develop Your Diffusing Skills

Based in the Washington, D.C., metropolitan area, Jamal Edmonds (see Figure 14-15) is an educator, master hairstylist, and owner and creative director of Lamaj in the City and Boutique Lamaj. You can visit Jamal at www.jamaledmonds.com and on Instagram at @lamajbackwards. He shares this tip.

"If I had to give any styling tip, it would be about the Art of Diffusing. A lot of consumers don't understand the importance of diffusing, or that there is a particular way that you should do it, depending on the desired results.

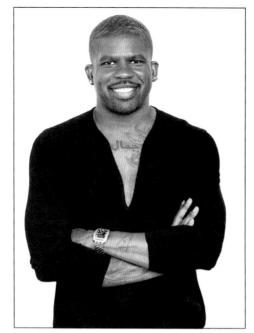

FIGURE 14-15:
Jamal
Edmonds,
owner and
creative
director of
Lamaj in
the City and
Boutique
Lamaj.

Photography by Antwan Maxwell

"For example, I always start with the *hovering* technique, which means that you hover the diffuser around your hair without touching it. This locks the curls in. If you want to reduce volume or collapse your curls, this is the perfect technique to do so. When my client's finished results require more work with encouraging or defining the natural curl pattern or creating volume, then I use the Diffuser Dance. You can do this for yourself when you want more volume. To do it, tilt your head all the way back and allow your curls to fall naturally. Then use the diffuser to move in and out or up and down. Once the back is about 50 percent dry, tilt your head to the right side and repeat. Then tilt your head to the left side, followed by the front of the head.

REMEMBER

"Always start diffusing with high heat and high wind. Once you are 60 percent dry, lower your heat and wind to avoid causing frizz. Also, always use your fingers while they are open for wet styling, but when drying or diffusing, keep the fingers closed and use a scrunching motion to help form the curls. This also helps avoid frizz. I promise this method for diffusing will give you more longevity with your wash-and-go's, and will also give you the curl definition you always wanted."

Chapter **15**

Ten Ways to Get Comfortable with Your Natural and Curly Hair

nfortunately, we don't all start off loving the hair that we're born with. In turn, figuring out how to wear our natural and curly hair with comfort and confidence can be a challenge. Even if you've worn your hair natural and curly for several years, you can still struggle with caring for it every now and then.

When you first decide to go natural, you may have some friends and family who don't know what that actually means, and they can bombard you with questions that might make you uncomfortable. They may say silly things such as, "But I love your hair more when it's straight." Please don't take it personally. I know that's a hard one, but most of the time, they don't know better, and you waste too much energy giving it any attention.

Everyone who has curly hair has their own hair story, and the more you feel comfortable expressing your story, the more everyone in your life accepts it.

Here's some good news: No matter what your hair's curl pattern, the natural hair community is positive and ready to embrace you and encourage you to say goodbye to unhealthy, chemically treated hair and hello to wearing your beautiful natural and curly hair.

But you might have to be a little uncomfortable to get comfortable. That's life, right? And I know if you're reading this book, you're definitely up for the challenge.

In this chapter, I give you ten tips to help you build confidence so that you can wear your beautiful natural and curly hair with pride.

Practice Self-Love

I know some people find practicing self-love difficult, but I'm a big proponent of it. Self-love can mean something different from person to person because you have so many different ways that you can take care of and love yourself.

To me, self-love means finding ways to support your physical, psychological, and spiritual well-being. Self-love is honoring your own desires, taking care of yourself, and not sacrificing to please or impress others. Self-love applies to all aspects of yourself, including your hair.

By figuring out what self-love looks like for you, not only can you get comfortable with your natural or curly hair, but you can also improve your mental wellness. Fully embracing and celebrating yourself is an important part of your hair journey. When you believe that every part of you is beautiful, you can truly express yourself fully.

Practicing self-love doesn't involve just your feelings; your actions also play a big part. Making time to take care of yourself in any way is an act of love. Devoting time and resources to caring for your hair to keep it healthy and happy is an enormous act of self-love. Sometimes, you may struggle to make yourself a priority in today's busy world, but I encourage you to do just that.

Take baby steps to avoid being overwhelmed. Give yourself a break from self-judgment and speak about yourself with love and kindness. Make yourself a priority and trust that you're doing the best you can do to take care of yourself. And don't forget to forgive yourself for those moments when you aren't so nice to yourself. Set boundaries to keep negative energy from yourself and from others at bay.

Commit to the Long Game

Your hair journey is a marathon, not a sprint. On average, hair grows only about a half an inch a month. So for people who are transitioning from relaxers, seeing what their natural texture has to offer takes a long time. Committing is the only way to give your natural and curly hair a chance to live up to its full potential.

Wrap your mind around the fact that this is a long game. Embracing the slow pace can help you manage expectations and celebrate the wins, no matter how small or incremental. Expect that days may come where you feel frustrated or tired of waiting. Then you may have days where you step back and notice the progress. Do your best to remind yourself that, even though it can feel like a long journey at times, it's one filled with discovery and surprises.

TIP

On the days it feels like your hair is growing at a slug's pace, do something that makes you feel happy or beautiful. Treat yourself and your hair right — you deserve it.

I promise you, after you reach a certain point in your natural hair Journey, you really start to enjoy the versatility.

Dare to Not Compare

Don't compare your curls to other curlies. Your hair journey is a personal one. What works for others might not work for you. Your hair makes you unique, and comparing your curls to your best friend's hair can only leave you lost and confused. We all have different hair types, textures, lifestyles, and habits.

Don't get me wrong; a fellow curl-friend might have some suggestions that can work for you. Just understand that those tips might not give you the results you want. But you only know for sure if you give them a try. The best way to get comfortable with your curls is to find out what works for you.

Also, if you have friends who are on their own hair journey, share with them what works for you, while supporting them when they try their own ideas. No one has a one-size-fits-all solution to any of this. Hair care and styling is a complex mix of science, art, and personality. Find your own hair expression, let others find theirs, and always celebrate each other!

Find a Good Hair Care Regimen

Regular hair care helps you get comfortable with your natural and curly hair. If you're good to your hair, your hair is good to you. Figuring out how to take care of your natural and curly hair takes time, but commit to figuring out your perfect daily, weekly, and monthly hair care regimen. Experiment with different products and tools. Discover what you can do yourself, and what you want a stylist to do for you. Then, after you find out what works for you, keep it going.

If you don't take care of your hair, you see and feel the difference, which inevitably decreases your comfort level with your curls. When you keep up with your hair regimen, your hair looks and stays healthy, which can help you feel comfortable and confident.

Wear Your Hair Out

When you first start transitioning to natural hair, it's normal to feel a little nervous and uncomfortable *wearing your hair out* (without any hair ties or bands to contain it), particularly at school and work, or around people who haven't see your natural texture. Just remember that you and your hair are beautiful.

Take baby steps at first if you need to — no need to rush, just ease into it. Start by wearing your hair out only on the weekends to build your confidence until you feel ready to rock your curls to work or school. Maybe even give yourself a self-love pep talk before you go out.

REMEMBER

Day one of wearing your hair out might feel weird because you might feel like everyone is looking at your hair. Trust me — they'll adjust. And it's not about them, anyway. It's about how you feel.

Experiment with Extensions

When you feel tired of waiting or need a change of hair scenery, expand your options with hair extensions! They are fun and interesting and can be super easy to install (or have a stylist install). Extensions can give you the volume and length you want while you're transitioning away from relaxer to your natural hair or during the in-between stage of your hair growing out fully to your desired length. You can find them as clip-ins for temporary use or bundles for the times that you want a sew-in for protective styling.

Extensions provide an especially fabulous option for folks who are used to or prefer long hair. If you're feeling too naked or exposed with your short hair, treat yourself to a shopping trip. At every step of your journey, do whatever you need to make yourself feel as good as possible. Make your hair journey a positive experience for you. The more you find ways to enjoy the journey and the more you can find solutions to the challenges, the more comfortable you feel with your natural hair. Head to Chapter 9 for more how-tos on extensions.

If you want to look into natural hair extensions, head over to one of my personal faves in the extension business, Knappy Hair Extensions. They have all hair textures, colors, and styles, and you can find one that matches yours perfectly. For more information, flip to Chapter 9.

Take the No-Heat Challenge

If you use heat to style your hair, listen up to this tip!

Take the no-heat challenge — give your hair an extended time without direct heat. Try doing this challenge for anywhere from two weeks to a year. How long you go totally depends on you and your hair goals. During this time, use low-manipulation and protective styles that don't require direct heat.

This challenge can help you see your natural hair texture and determine what works best for it. Full disclosure: This tip may actually make you feel less comfortable with your natural hair at first, but that's only because it's something new (it's not called a challenge for nothing!). But stick with it, and you absolutely will get comfortable with your hair.

Although there's nothing wrong with heat styling every now and then, you're never going to get comfortable with your curls if you don't resist the urge to straighten them all the time.

Expand Your Education

We all know that knowledge is power, and that idea applies to natural hair care. From products to tools (visit Chapters 7 and 8 for more on those) and accessories, the natural hair community continues to evolve daily. Staying on top of what's new, now, and next can help you keep your curls in tip-top shape and your confidence on high.

You can feel overwhelmed sometimes when you try to absorb all of this information, especially because it seems to change rapidly. But don't get discouraged. Just focus on one thing at a time. Maybe one week, you focus on understanding more about wash day. Maybe another week, you devote yourself to figuring out braiding. And some other time, you take a peek at what new combs and brushes are on the market.

This book can give you a great start because it has a little bit of everything. But I encourage you to always stay hungry for more hair knowledge. Go out and get it in the ways that work for you, whether that means reading magazines, browsing the web, scrolling social media, consulting with a professional stylist, or chatting with your friends at the salon.

REMEMBER

You don't have to know everything about everything. In fact, you can't. Even one new nugget of information gives you enough to keep your brain (and hair) growing.

Find a Feel-Good Community

Your natural hair journey is more than just improving the health of your hair; it's also about nurturing your positive feelings and thoughts towards your natural hair.

The natural and curly hair movement has come a long way, and more celebrities are wearing their natural hair in television, movies, and other media. You might find it helpful to follow people on social media who post images and videos that show themselves embracing and loving their natural hair.

Surround yourself with like-minded people. Find a salon where you feel welcomed and happy. Hang out with other folks who rock their natural hair without apology. Find people who enjoy experimenting with their braid, locs, afros, and twist outs. These are your hair role models! The more time you can spend with them personally or enjoy the media that they produce, the more positive their effect on you. Their enthusiasm, skills, and hair love can inspire you to love your own hair.

TIP

If any people in your life or any social media apps make you feel negatively about your hair, consider reducing or eliminating the time and space that you give to them. Make room for those who support your journey.

Pick Patience

Have fun and be patient with yourself. Whenever I think of natural and curly hair, the word "carefree" comes to mind. Have fun creating a new image of yourself and telling a different story. Push past the anxiety and focus on all the exciting things happening in your life. The new products and tools, and the plethora of new styles to try, make this journey even more exciting. Of course, you have to deal with some trial and error because change doesn't happen overnight. It takes time. Be patient and allow yourself to enjoy the process because — at the end of the day — it's just hair.

REMEMBER

The world is yours, baby, you got the power — CURLPOWER!

Index

blowing out hair, 179–182

general discussion, 141–146

maintaining healthy hair, 96–97

overview, 18

using on wash day, 70

drying hair

brushes for, 130, 132–133

methods for, 68–70

for twist outs, 194

before using blow dryer, 142

in winter, 93

durags, 100

Dyson Supersonic hair dryer, 142–143

E

early childhood, hair care in. *See* child-friendly styles; children

eczema (atopic dermatitis), 26–27

edge control, 19, 123, 155

Edmonds, Jamal, 255–256

education, expanding, 261–262

elasticity

defined, 14

determining, 29–30

electric hot combs, 146–147

emollients, 110–111, 112–113

environment, effect on hair

humectant performance and, 112

humidity, 90–91

overview, 88, 89

pollution, 89

seasonal change, 91–93

essential oils, 119

exercise, 241

exfoliation, scalp, 27

expert styling tips

detangling, 250–251

diffusing, 255–256

double conditioning, stopping, 247–248

hair loss, combating with keratin fibers, 244–247

hydrate, trim, and have fun, 253–254

overview, 243–244

protective styles, 252–253

sealing cuticle with leave-in conditioner, 249–250

steam, using to improve absorption, 254–255

twist outs, 248–249

wash-and-go, mastering, 251–252

extensions

clip-in, 167–169

experimenting with, 260–261

favorites, 171–172

lock, 166

overview, 166–167

scalp care when using, 191

sew-in, 169–170

textures, 188–191

types of, 187

F

fabric covered bands, 218, 226

fall wigs, 172

fatty alcohols, 118

faux locs, 166, 186, 190, 191

Felicia Leatherwood detangler brush, 131

fine hair, 37, 40

fine-tooth combs, 18, 135–136, 213

finger detangling, 55

finger twist, 83

fingers, styling with, 63–65

flat irons

general discussion, 140–141

overview, 18

safe use of, 97

sealing ends of braids with, 192–193

flat twists, 82, 163, 194–195

flaxseed gel, 128

flexible curling rods (flexi-rods), 47, 48

follicle, hair, 24–25

fragrances, 118–119

freeform locking technique, 164

French braid, 160

hairstylists. *See also* expert styling tips
  bringing children to, 219, 222, 232
  cutting hair with, 178
  finding, 102–103, 181
  overview, 13, 100–101
  permanent hair coloring and bleaching, 177
  questions to ask, 103–104
  reasons to consult with, 101–102
half wigs, 172
hard water, 89
Havana twists, 186
head wraps, 202–203
headbands, 229–230
health, focusing on, 241
healthy hair
  bad hair days, 86
  color-treated hair, 98–99
  environment, effect of, 89–93
  as foundation of achieving any hairstyle, 81
  as good hair, 35
  hairstylists, consulting with, 100–104
  heat styling, 96–98
  low-manipulation techniques, 95–96
  moisturizing, 86–88
  nighttime accessories, 99–100
  overview, 85
  trimming hair, 94–95
heat protectants, 92, 99, 126, 139
heat styling
  avoiding excessive, 74, 239–240
  blow dryers, 141–146
  curling iron or wand, 147–148
  flat iron, 140–141
  and hair texture, 37, 38
  healthy hair tips, 96–98
  hot combs, 146–147
  and humidity, 91
  and moisture of hair, 88
  no-heat challenge, 261
  overview, 18, 139

Type 2 hair maintenance, 40
  when transitioning, 47
high density hair, 44
high elasticity, 30
high porosity hair, 28–29
honey, 127
hooded dryers, 96–97, 146
hot combs (pressing combs), 18, 146–147
hot oil treatments, 66, 124–126
hot water, sealing ends of braids with, 192
hovering technique, 256
human hair extensions, 187
humectants, 60, 86–87, 110–112
humidity, 90–91, 112
hydrating shampoo, 120–121
hydration
  in afro maintenance, 199
  checking hair's level of, 109–110
  expert tips for, 253–254
  overview, 108–109
  role in health, 241
  vital hair care ingredients, 110–112

I

icons, explained, 3
in-between stage, navigating, 50, 73
infancy, hair care in. *See* kids
interlocking, 165–166

J

Janelle, Keandra, 171
Jheri curl, 86
Johnson, Evie, 250–251
jojoba oil, 125

K

keratin, 114, 244–247
kid-friendly styles
  afros and puffs, 227, 229–230

choosing, 124–126

hot oil treatments, 66, 124–126

for keeping twists fresh, 195

LOC method, 88, 99, 195, 217

for moisturizing, 88

overview, 19

for summer use, 92

for Type 3 hair, 41

olive oil, 125

organic silicones, 117

over-manipulation of hair, avoiding, 240

P

paddle brushes, 132–133

palm rolling, 166

parabens, 116–117

parents, attitude toward hair, 207, 208–209, 211, 214. *See also* child-friendly styles; children

patience, importance of, 262–263

peppermint oil, 57, 128

permanent hair coloring and bleaching, 177

physical effects of hair, 22

pineappling, 77–78, 195

plaits. *See* braids

plopping, 69

pollution, 89

ponytails, 225–226

porosity

defined, 14

determining, 28–29, 88

and hydration, 108

praying hands method, 64

prejudice, 8–11

pressing combs (hot combs), 18, 146–147

products. *See also specific products*

based on porosity, 29

for children, 216, 233

for color-treated hair, 98

for co-washing, 122

creating your own, 127–128

for daily use, selecting, 75

experimenting with, 73

for handling humidity, 90

heat protectants, 139

ingredients doubling as supplements, 114–115

ingredients to avoid, 115–119

for moisturizing, 87–88

for morning routine, 79–80

for nighttime routine, 76

overview, 17–19, 107–108

pollution, protecting against, 89

seeing professional for help with, 101

for summer use, 92

for Type 2 hair maintenance, 40

for Type 3 hair maintenance, 41

for Type 4 hair maintenance, 43

vital ingredients, 110–114

water as essential ingredient, 108–110

when transitioning, 47

professional hairstylists. *See also* expert styling tips

bringing children to, 219, 222, 232

cutting hair with, 178

finding, 102–103, 181

overview, 13, 100–101

permanent hair coloring and bleaching, 177

questions to ask, 103–104

reasons to consult with, 101–102

protective styles. *See also* braids; extensions; twists; wigs

for children, 217, 218, 223

combating over-manipulation with, 240

expert tips for, 252–253

giving hair break from styling, 83

handling humidity, 91

for nighttime routine, 77–78

overview, 17, 20, 152

trying out, 74

when transitioning, 49

summer, effect on hair, 92
surface (rinse-out) conditioners, 60, 63, 124, 248
synthetic crochet hair extensions, 187, 192
synthetic fragrances, 118–119
systemic discrimination, 8–11

T

TA (traction alopecia), 155, 219, 226, 244
taping wigs, 176
Tarrant, Jacqueline, 244–247
tea tree oil, 57, 128, 238
Technical Stuff icon, explained, 3
telogen (rest) phase, 32, 33
texture, hair
  attitudes toward, changes in, 10
  in biracial and multiracial children, 213–214
  in children, 215
  coarse hair, 38
  defined, 15, 36
  fine hair, 37
  identifying, 36–38
  medium hair, 37
  relation to follicle, 24–25
textured hair. See natural and curly hair
three-strand twists, 194
Tip icon, explained, 3
titanium plates, flat irons with, 140
toddlerhood, hair care in. See child-friendly styles; children
tools. See also blow dryers; brushes; combs
  for braiding, 154
  for children, 213
  curling irons or wands, 18, 97, 147–148
  for detangling hair, 55, 56
  experimenting with, 74
  flat irons, 18, 97, 140–141, 192–193
  hooded dryers, 96–97, 146
  hot combs, 18, 146–147
  for morning routine, 79–80
  overview, 17–19, 129
tourmaline plates, flat irons with, 140

traction alopecia (TA), 155, 219, 226, 244
transition (catagen) phase, 32, 33
transitioning
  defined, 14
  seeing professional for, 101
  tips for, 46–49
trauma, hair-related, 7, 11–12, 211, 214, 222
trichologists, 45
trimming hair
  expert tips for, 253–254
  importance of, 239
  role in healthy hair, 81–82, 94–95
  seeing professional for, 101
  Type 2 hair, 40
  Type 3 hair, 41
  Type 4 hair, 43
  when transitioning, 47
t-shirt, drying hair with, 69
turbans, styling hair with, 202–203
twist outs
  crochet, 186
  defined, 14, 161
  expert tips for, 248–249
  keeping fresh between wash days, 195
  nighttime routine, 77
  overview, 194–195
twisted extensions, 190
twisting creams, 122
twists. See also twist outs
  for children, 226–227
  comb, 82
  finger, 83
  flat, 82, 163, 194–195
  Havana, 186
  overview, 161, 193
  playing around with, 82–83
  Senegalese, 163, 164, 186, 189
  styling options, 193–195
  three-strand, 194
  two-strand, 82, 161–162, 166
two-strand twists, 82, 161–162, 166

About the Author

A celebrity hairstylist with over 30 years of experience, **Johnny Wright** is no stranger to success. He was born and raised on the south side of Chicago and got his start in the styling world as a child watching his grandmother do press-and-curls on the back porch.

After working his way through Chicago and then Los Angeles, he spent eight years as Michelle Obama's personal hairstylist during the Obama Administration. Since 2019, he's worked as Tamron Hall's key hairstylist on her Emmy Award–winning eponymous daytime talk show and most recently co-starred in *To Catch a Beautician* with Tamar Braxton on VH1. You can also see his work on celebrities such as Queen Latifah, Kerry Washington, Tiffany Cross, Angela Rye, and Samira Wiley, to name a few.

His career spans professional and artistic achievements such as acting as creative director for SoftSheen-Carson (a L'Oreal product line), making HSN appearances, conducting brand ambassadorships, and receiving industry awards. Johnny's unique success is owed in part to years of welcoming all hair textures and types to his chair and developing master styling skills and precision cutting techniques, as well as his passion for education, business ingenuity, and infectious upbeat personality.

Dedication

I dedicate this book to my personal trinity:

My late grandmother, Minnie Brown, who was an amazing hairstylist and let me sit at her feet on the porch watching her do hair when I was 3 years old, and who still inspires me to this day.

My mother, Vernita T Wright, who was my first client and guinea pig, who never said no to any hairstyle I wanted to try, and gave me her gifts of humor and optimism that have made a world of difference to my career.

My dad, Edward Wright, Sr., who accepted me fully for who I was and single-handedly built me that salon in the basement on the south side of Chicago when I was just 14 years old, beginning my life as an entrepreneur.

You will always and forever be my heroes, and I cannot thank you enough.

Author's Acknowledgments

I would like to acknowledge and thank all of the people who have helped me through this process. Your efforts and generosity have been invaluable and so appreciated, and every one of you has a piece of my heart: my agent Nikita Adams; Tamron Hall and *The Tamron Hall Show*; the Wiley editorial team, including Sarah Sypniewski, Tracy Boggier, Donna Wright, and Laura K. Miller; technical editor Veronique Morrison; the models Eugenia Washington, Lauren Wilkins, Jared Grange, and Alexis Willis; my photographer Wardell Malloy and crowdMGMT; photo assistant Tevin Baker; production assistant Jaden; Mikayla Miller and Maria Troncoso de Gibbs (Digitech); my makeup artist Mila Thomas; my assistants Lizzie Levine and Liz; the featured experts Jacqueline Tarrant, Monica Stevens, Larry J. Sims, Tippi Shorter Rank, Evie Johnson, Ursula Stephens, Nicole Mangrum, Tym Wallace, Kim Kimble, and Jamal Edmonds; my supporters RevAir, Sally Beauty, and KJ Sandifer (the founder of KnappyHair Extensions); my marketing team India and Michelle; and my dear friends and family Holly, Sir John, LaToiya (a.k.a. Tata), Brandi, Reena Patton, and Norell Giancana.

Very special thanks to Michelle Obama and all of my amazing clients for being such a big part of this ongoing journey. You know who you are.

Publisher's Acknowledgments

Senior Acquisitions Editor: Tracy Boggier

Contributor: Sarah Sypniewski

Project Editor: Donna Wright

Copy Editor: Laura K. Miller

Technical Editor: Veronique Morrison

Proofreader: Debbye Butler

Photographer: Wardell Malloy,
    unless otherwise noted

Illustrator: Rashell Smith

Production Editor: Mohammed Zafar Ali

Cover Images: front: © Wardell Malloy with
    crowdMGMT; back: © Paethegee Inc/Getty
    Images; Courtesy of Michael Letterlough, Jr.

Take dummies with you everywhere you go!

Whether you are excited about e-books, want more from the web, must have your mobile apps, or are swept up in social media, dummies makes everything easier.

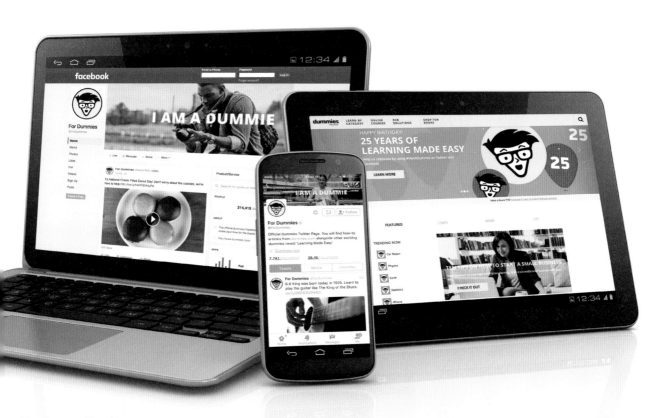

Find us online!

dummies.com

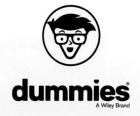

Leverage the power

Dummies is the global leader in the reference category and one of the most trusted and highly regarded brands in the world. No longer just focused on books, customers now have access to the dummies content they need in the format they want. Together we'll craft a solution that engages your customers, stands out from the competition, and helps you meet your goals.

Advertising & Sponsorships

Connect with an engaged audience on a powerful multimedia site, and position your message alongside expert how-to content. Dummies.com is a one-stop shop for free, online information and know-how curated by a team of experts.

- Targeted ads
- Video
- Email Marketing

- Microsites
- Sweepstakes sponsorship

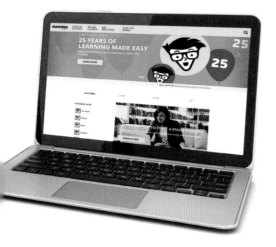

20 MILLION
PAGE VIEWS
EVERY SINGLE MONTH

15 MILLION
UNIQUE
VISITORS PER MONTH

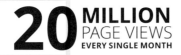

43%
OF ALL VISITORS
ACCESS THE SITE
VIA THEIR MOBILE DEVICES

700,000 NEWSLETTER
SUBSCRIPTIONS
TO THE INBOXES OF
300,000 UNIQUE INDIVIDUALS
EVERY WEEK

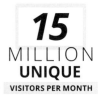

# of dummies

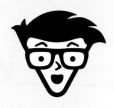

Custom Publishing

Reach a global audience in any language by creating a solution that will differentiate you from competitors, amplify your message, and encourage customers to make a buying decision.

- Apps
- Books
- eBooks
- Video
- Audio
- Webinars

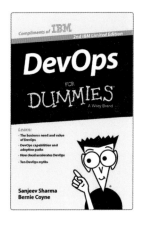
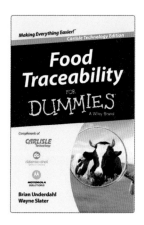
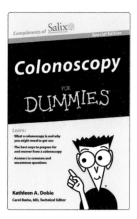
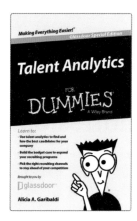

Brand Licensing & Content

Leverage the strength of the world's most popular reference brand to reach new audiences and channels of distribution.

For more information, visit dummies.com/biz

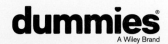

PERSONAL ENRICHMENT

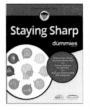
9781119187790
USA $26.00
CAN $31.99
UK £19.99

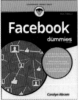
9781119179030
USA $21.99
CAN $25.99
UK £16.99

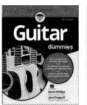
9781119293354
USA $24.99
CAN $29.99
UK £17.99

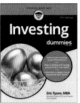
9781119293347
USA $22.99
CAN $27.99
UK £16.99

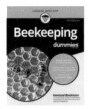
9781119310068
USA $22.99
CAN $27.99
UK £16.99

9781119235606
USA $24.99
CAN $29.99
UK £17.99

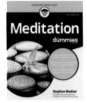
9781119251163
USA $24.99
CAN $29.99
UK £17.99

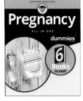
9781119235491
USA $26.99
CAN $31.99
UK £19.99

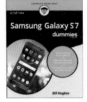
9781119279952
USA $24.99
CAN $29.99
UK £17.99

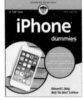
9781119283133
USA $24.99
CAN $29.99
UK £17.99

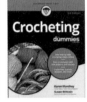
9781119287117
USA $24.99
CAN $29.99
UK £16.99

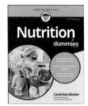
9781119130246
USA $22.99
CAN $27.99
UK £16.99

PROFESSIONAL DEVELOPMENT

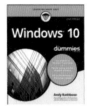
9781119311041
USA $24.99
CAN $29.99
UK £17.99

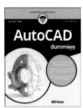
9781119255796
USA $39.99
CAN $47.99
UK £27.99

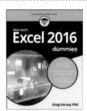
9781119293439
USA $26.99
CAN $31.99
UK £19.99

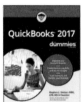
9781119281467
USA $26.99
CAN $31.99
UK £19.99

9781119280651
USA $29.99
CAN $35.99
UK £21.99

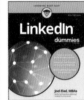
9781119251132
USA $24.99
CAN $29.99
UK £17.99

9781119310563
USA $34.00
CAN $41.99
UK £24.99

9781119181705
USA $29.99
CAN $35.99
UK £21.99

9781119263593
USA $26.99
CAN $31.99
UK £19.99

9781119257769
USA $29.99
CAN $35.99
UK £21.99

9781119293477
USA $26.99
CAN $31.99
UK £19.99

9781119265313
USA $24.99
CAN $29.99
UK £17.99

9781119239314
USA $29.99
CAN $35.99
UK £21.99

9781119293323
USA $29.99
CAN $35.99
UK £21.99

dummies.com

dummies®
A Wiley Brand